Dr Carmel Harrington (PhD, LLB, BSc, DipEd) has been working in the world of sleep for nearly 20 years.

A former lawyer and educator, she has a PhD in Sleep Medicine from the University of Sydney and consults to companies and educational institutions on sleep health both locally and overseas.

Dr Harrington is the Managing Director of 'Sleep for Health' and an Honorary Research Fellow at the Children's Hospital, Westmead. She is a founding member of the Sleep Health Foundation and a member of the Australasian Sleep Association.

In 2012 Dr Harrington published her first book, *The Sleep Diet*, which explained the fundamental connection between sleep and wellness, particularly highlighting how sleep impacts on our ability to maintain a healthy body weight.

www.sleepforhealth.com.au

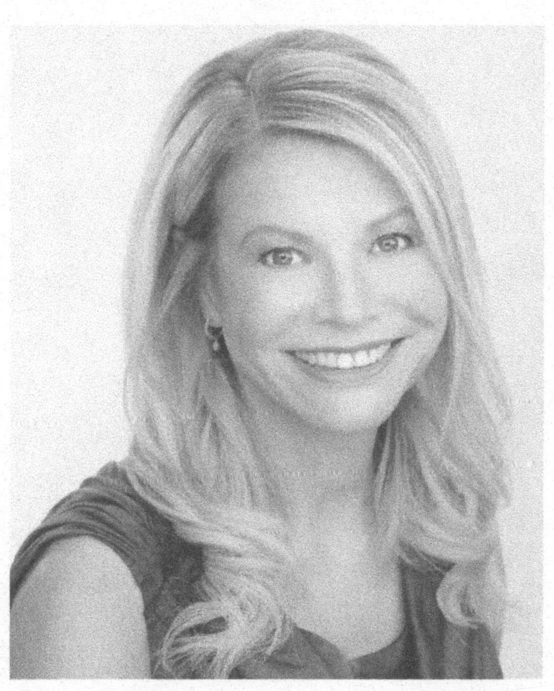

Also by Carmel Harrington

The Sleep Diet

The Complete Guide to a Good Night's Sleep

Dr Carmel Harrington
Australian Sleep Expert

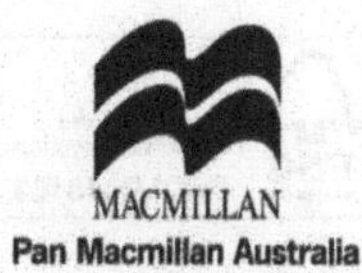

MACMILLAN
Pan Macmillan Australia

Some of the people in this book have had their
names changed to protect their identities

First published 2014 in Macmillan by Pan Macmillan Australia Pty Ltd
1 Market Street, Sydney, New South Wales, Australia, 2000

Cataloguing-in-Publication entry is available
from the National Library of Australia
http://catalogue.nla.gov.au

Typeset in Adobe Caslon Pro by Midland Typesetters, Australia
Printed by IVE
Internal text design by fisheye design group
Index by Trevor Matthews

It is recommended that individually tailored advice is sought
from your healthcare professional.

The author and the publisher have made every effort to contact copyright holders for material used in this book. Any person or organisation that may have been overlooked should contact the publisher.

For

Steven,

&

Alexander, Charlotte and Damien

Contents

Introduction

'Sleep . . . Balm of hurt minds, great nature's second course,
Chief nourisher in life's feast.'

Shakespeare (*Macbeth*, Act 2, Scene 2)

ALTHOUGH THESE WORDS WERE WRITTEN over four hundred years ago, they are as true today as they were then. In our current too-busy world many of us have almost forgotten what a good night's sleep feels like. We may feel like it has been forever since we were able to go to bed, sleep and simply wake up 8 hours later with little memory of the intervening hours. We may long for those days when we woke feeling energised and invigorated, looking forward to the challenges of the day. We may even have developed a sense of despair in our ability to ever sleep well again.

If some or all of this describes your attitude towards sleep then I am pleased that you have picked up this book. I am confident that as you read through the following chapters and learn about the processes of sleep and begin to understand how to manage them, your negative feelings will dissipate. You will gradually rediscover the joy of sleep and once again experience the delight of being nourished and refreshed by sleeping eight uninterrupted hours.

When we can't sleep and are still awake at 3 am after tossing and turning for hours, we may think that we are the only ones suffering the exhaustion of sleeplessness. This is far from reality and it seems that more and more people are finding sleep increasingly elusive. Research from the US indicates that annually more than 35% of adults suffer sleeplessness symptoms.

Part of the problem is that these days we have so much to do and so much going on around us that we often don't pay much attention to sleep – instead, we live our lives much like the White Rabbit in *Alice in Wonderland*. Always rushing from place to place, feeling constantly like we are running late, might work for a while but, for many of us, there will come a time when maintaining this pace is not sustainable – we may begin to suffer ill-health, we may find we have lost our motivation, and we may feel depressed or just exhausted. There are many reasons why we start to evaluate the way we live our life and at times like these, we may well start to think about the role sleep plays in how we think and feel.

If you are reading this book then chances are you have recognised the importance of sleep and want to do something about your sleeping pattern. This is a great first step. I find it very interesting that so often discussions about our physical and psychological well-being centre only on our nutrition and our exercise without mentioning our sleep. Yet sleep is fundamental to how well we are able to live our lives, and if nutrition and exercise are perceived as two pillars of health then sleep needs to be considered our third pillar.

Many of us already understand that sleep is integral to our health – but try as we might we are just not able to achieve the sleep that we know is so necessary for our vitality. For us, our bed has become a battlefield where, instead of experiencing deep slumber, we all too often toss and turn, feeling frustrated, exhausted and even perhaps a sense of helplessness at our inability to sleep, until eventually there is an acceptance that soon, with only a few hours of sleep, we will get up and face a new day. This would be bad enough if it were to happen once or twice a month but for many people it goes on night after night, week after week and year after year.

When we can't sleep, life can become extremely difficult. Sleep is meant to be our time for refreshment and restoration. It is an opportunity, as Shakespeare said, for our minds and bodies to be 'nourished', so that when we wake we are enthusiastic and ready to enjoy the pleasures and to manage the stresses of our life. Without sleep, however, simple tasks and challenges can quickly become insurmountable and our relationships suffer.

So how did this happen? How did sleep become so difficult for so many of us? To understand the reasons behind this we need to realise that there is a major difference between the idea that sleep is natural and the idea that sleep should come naturally to us.

Deep, restful sleep relies upon a whole series of interlocking biological processes. If these processes do not work in harmony then we will not be able to get to sleep or to maintain sleep. While these biological processes have been highly effective in giving humans good sleep for millennia, in recent times we have unknowingly sabotaged our ability to sleep, so that right now we are seeing a serious problem with sleeplessness and its consequent health and relationship problems.

We seem to have put aside the fact that sleep nourishes us. We have filled our world with so much light, noise and activity that sleep has become unnaturally difficult. Somewhere along the way, many of us have become too much like the White Rabbit and lost the ability (or the time) to switch off sufficiently to allow sleep to happen. Without switching off, deep, restful sleep will be elusive.

This book is about learning how to access the off-switch again. Many books about overcoming sleeplessness rely on general solutions that apply to everyone. But, just as there are particular foods that are just right for you and specific exercises that suit you best, so too are there sleep solutions that are right just for you.

Sleep solutions are not one-size-fits-all. Sleep is highly individual and there are many reasons why we may not be sleeping well. I have been working in the world of sleep for almost 20 years now and I have met many people with a wide variety of sleeping difficulties. Throughout this book we are going to meet some of these people and learn about their sleep problems and how these problems manifested in real life. We will learn how they managed to overcome their particular sleep difficulties and discover the processes they implemented in order to do this. It is by understanding these different problems and their various solutions that we will gain an insight into our own particular sleep issues and learn how to manage our sleep so that we are able to achieve good sleep on a regular basis.

In order for us to have deep, restful sleep a number of things need to happen. Firstly, we need to understand the processes of sleep and its patterns. Once we understand this it will be possible to discover why *you*, as an individual, are not sleeping well. When this is established it is then possible to uncover what in particular enhances your sleep, and then to start to manipulate the various sleep processes so that you are able to have deep, restful sleep on a regular basis.

This book is a journey through sleep and it tackles problems progressively. Many of us are tempted to dip in and out of a book like this, seeking out and reading only those bits that we think are particularly relevant to our problem. For example, we may be experiencing long-term trouble trying to get to sleep and so we may decide to go straight to the chapter dealing with this. To completely overcome your sleep difficulties though it's best to follow this journey in the order that it is presented in this book. By doing this you will be able to fully understand sleep, see where your problem lies and, importantly, how it can be solved.

All of this will take time and effort, but it will be worth it. When the reason for your sleeplessness is discovered it can be treated, and when treated you will rediscover refreshing and invigorating sleep. You will once again experience the joy of sleep and the wondrous nourishing feeling of waking after a long and contented (and undisturbed) sleep.

Sleep is our third pillar of health. It is as important as good nutrition and exercise If we take away one of the pillars our physical and psychological well-being will bear the consequences.

So, let's get started . . .

Chapter 1

Understanding the problem

THE IMPORTANCE OF SLEEP WAS recognised as far back as the time of the ancient Greeks and Romans. These civilisations had numerous powerful sleep gods, such as Hypnos, Somnus and Morpheus, and it is from these ancient times that such words as 'hypnotic' (to describe a sleep-inducing drug), 'somnolent' (to describe the state of drowsiness) and 'morphine' are derived.

We know that even in these early times, long before the electric light and the internet, people experienced problems with sleep because the use of sleeping aids such as valerian, chamomile and the poppy flower is well documented. The word to describe sleeplessness, 'insomnia', comes from the Latin *in* (meaning not) and *somnus* (meaning sleep) and was first used by modern medicine around the beginning of the 17th century to describe the inability to sleep.

Today, insomnia is used to describe the situation when someone has difficulty falling asleep and/or staying asleep, and consequently experiences some daytime impairment, such as excessive tiredness, mood changes or lack of energy. Basically someone will be described as having insomnia if they cannot get adequate sleep. While we use only one word to describe this situation – insomnia – we should not make the mistake of thinking that there is only one cause. There are numerous types of insomnia and many causes.

Insomnia is the most common of all sleep disorders and is estimated to affect at least one in three people at some stage of their lives. It can affect all of us, no matter how old or young we are.

Most insomnia only persists for a night or two, but sometimes it will last for weeks, months or even years.

Anyone who has experienced even brief bouts of sleeplessness lasting more than one or two nights knows just how debilitating a few nights of restricted sleep can be. After getting too little sleep for a few days we begin to feel excessively tired, cranky, depressed, unmotivated, indecisive and unable to learn or process information well. We also invariably feel disinclined to exercise or participate in activity. When we do not get enough sleep there is a deregulation of our appetite hormones so we are also very hungry and have a strong desire to eat all the wrong types of food – like chocolate, chips and hamburgers.

Imagine then, how much more these feelings are exacerbated when a person gets 5–6 hours' sleep per night three or more times each week over months and perhaps even years. These people truly suffer and they would gladly give almost anything for a good night's sleep.

Frequently, one of the first steps in the process of overcoming sleeplessness is to classify the type of insomnia being experienced. There are a number of ways this can be done but often it is described either as 'transient', lasting anywhere from 1–2 nights to a few weeks, or 'chronic' when the insomnia has persisted for more than 6 months.

While this may be a convenient medical division, for people suffering from sleeplessness the categorisation can be artificial as they may experience repeated episodes of transient insomnia over a period of many years. In situations like these, even though the insomnia would be correctly diagnosed as transient, it is more akin to chronic insomnia as these episodes can be just as distressing as the experience of someone who has struggled with sleep consistently over an extended period of time.

All of us would have had at least one bad night, or even a few bad nights, of sleep due to some stress or disruption to our routine. The reason for the wakefulness is usually apparent and self-limiting. For example, if the difficulty sleeping was caused by an anxiety over an exam, once the exam is completed then normal sleep usually returns. While this is distressing for the days or the week that the bad sleep persists it is generally manageable and short-lived. If a few days or a week of insomnia turns into a month of sleeplessness, however, then this becomes a real problem.

A typical example of this is sometimes seen when a person experiences a traumatic event in their life, such as a relationship break-up. At such times it is common for people to experience difficulty sleeping, often only getting about 4–5 hours per night. As a result they feel not only emotionally wrought, but also desperately tired. Due to this tiredness they may start to develop some unhealthy sleep habits, which makes sleep even harder to come by. If these bad sleep habits are not cut short then it is likely that what should have been a brief bout of sleeplessness ends up lasting much longer and causing havoc to their well-being.

When a person cannot sleep well for a few weeks they will often seek out a sleeping aid. Sleeping aids fall broadly into two categories – self-prescribed or medically prescribed. Self-prescribed aids, referred to as self-medication, include alcohol or illicit drugs, such as marijuana, or over-the-counter medications such as antihistamines, some pain killers or herbal preparations. Medically prescribed sleeping aids are commonly known as sleeping pills. In some cases, these may be an antidepressant with sleepiness as a side-effect.

While a sleeping aid during times of transient insomnia may provide much needed relief and be very effective in achieving sleep, it is important to always use such medications with caution. If care is not taken people can become dependent on the use of the sleeping aid, either physically or emotionally. It is not recommended that sleeping aids be taken any longer than 3–4 weeks.

While transient insomnia impacts significantly on a person's health and well-being, the most serious type of insomnia is the chronic form. A person is considered to be suffering from chronic insomnia if they have been experiencing sleeplessness and its negative effects for more than 6 months. The person suffering from chronic insomnia will usually have developed a myriad of coping strategies that they have come to rely on over the years, which continue the cycle of poor sleep.

Unlike transient insomnia, where it is often easy to detect the cause and effect, in chronic insomnia it is generally difficult to discern when and how the problem started. In many instances, in fact, this will never be known. However, in terms of chronic insomnia, how or when it started becomes irrelevant and what is most important is unravelling the current reason for the sleeplessness.

Research into the consequences of chronic insomnia paints a grim picture. Population studies of insomnia have shown that it has both short-term and long-term effects. If you are reading this book and are currently suffering from lack of sleep these consequences will come as no surprise.

When we do not sleep well our mood is affected – and not to our advantage. A bad night of sleep will invariably result in a poor mood state which will include such characteristics as grumpiness, a short temper, intolerance and a general lack of motivation. All of which cannot help but have an impact on our relationships, both personal and professional. Not only are we generally in a bad mood after poor sleep but we are also less inclined to want to exercise and to participate in general activities. This lack of energy directly affects our sex drive, which also decreases as a consequence of sleeplessness.

Jack's story

Jack had not slept well in years. Occasionally he had times where he slept not too badly, but rarely would a week go by when he did not have at least one night where his sleep was truly awful. Over the years he had tried a variety of techniques to help him sleep but most had minimal effect. He had come to accept that he either had to live with his sleeplessness or take a sleeping pill – which he occasionally did when he really needed a good night's sleep. Mostly he resisted the sleeping pills because they left him feeling 'foggy' the next day. By and large, Jack considered he managed his sleeplessness not too badly.

Jack's wife, however, did not think he was managing his sleeplessness very well at all. It seemed to her that most of the time he was incredibly irritable and, while in the past this irritability seemed mostly concerned with his work, he now seemed irritable almost all the time. This was starting to have a real impact on his family life. He always seemed annoyed about something and when anything went awry, no matter how minor, he would invariably end up yelling at someone.

Jack saw absolutely no association between his sleepless nights and his anger and relationship problems. He was annoyed with his wife when she insisted that he talk to someone about it.

When I first met Jack he steadfastly maintained that while he knew he had problems sleeping he was able to manage them. Sure, he was sleepy, and if I could help with that, that would be good, but otherwise it wasn't a problem. He did admit that these days he was often irritable or angry but, he was quick to add, this was a result of his work colleagues, friends and family being variously incompetent, non-supportive or downright lazy and he was constantly having to solve one problem or another. His irritable mood, according to him, was definitely not a result of his sleeplessness.

When pressed a little further he mentioned that he and his wife were also having a few relationship problems. Not only did they seem to argue a lot these days, over relatively minor issues, but he also had no interest in sex and this was becoming a big issue between the two of them.

It took Jack some time to be convinced that many of the problems he was facing, including his decreased sex drive, could well be the consequence of his insomnia. By working out what was causing this and treating it, many, if not all his problems would either disappear or improve considerably. Once Jack was ready to accept that not only did his lack of sleep cause his sleepiness, it also impacted significantly on his good health, good mood and energy levels, he was also able to see just why he was so often annoyed and irritated with those around him and why he had lost interest in sex.

This realisation was a really important step as it motivated Jack to look further into what was causing his sleeplessness. As it turned out, Jack had undiagnosed restless legs – a sleep disorder that severely affects a person's ability to maintain sleep – and once this was treated Jack was able to get at least 7 hours of consolidated sleep most nights.

Not surprisingly, Jack's life turned around, almost overnight. He no longer felt annoyed by minor problems and was far less likely to lose his temper. Most importantly his family life was more harmonious and he and his wife were getting on far better than they had in years – and both were very happy that they could enjoy sex again.

As if the negative mood consequences were not enough, lack of sleep also directly affects our ability to learn and to think. In a sleep-deprived state it has been shown time and again that we become poor decision-makers, we are much more likely to make mistakes and our ability to learn is seriously impaired. An interesting and important study in this regard, involving over 1500 full-time university students aged 17 to 25 years of age, found that sleep quality and duration were among the main predictors of academic performance – the better the sleep the better the performance.

While the negative impacts on mood and thinking are considerable, a far greater and more serious problem of sleeplessness is the increased likelihood of an occupational or motor vehicle accident. Studies show that people with sleeping problems are seven times more likely to be involved in such accidents. Indeed, some of the more famous occupational disasters such as the Air France crash in 2009, the Chernobyl nuclear plant disaster, the Exxon Valdez oil spill and the Space Shuttle *Challenger* explosion have been found to be a direct result of operator fatigue.

While the short-term consequences of sleeplessness are well recognised by anyone who suffers from them, the long-term consequences of unresolved insomnia may come as a surprise. People suffering from chronic insomnia are far more likely to develop depression; certain types of cancer; cardiovascular diseases, such as high blood pressure and heart disease; and metabolic diseases, such as type 2 diabetes and obesity. These consequences of sleeplessness may be overwhelming but I mention them here because it is critically important that we know about them and are aware of the damage that ongoing sleeplessness can have on our health, well-being and relationships. If we realise these serious consequences we are far more likely to be that little bit more determined to work on our sleeping problems. For some it will take both time and effort to improve their sleep but, given the alternatives, it will be time and energy well spent.

This book offers a systematic approach to discover the basis of your nightly battle with sleep. It is important that you assume nothing because only by having an open mind will you be able to unmask the cause for your sleeplessness and then treat it.

A word of caution

Some of you may find the work you need to do to get your sleep in order difficult, especially when you are already feeling tired and unmotivated. You may be tempted to keep taking your sleeping pills. You are not alone. Research shows that an estimated 6–10% of adults take prescribed sleeping pills. But this is certainly not without its risks and you would be well advised to try to avoid this path.

A large US study published in 2012 evaluated more than 10,000 patients who received sleeping pill prescriptions and followed them for 2.5 years comparing their health outcomes to over 23,000 people who received no such prescriptions. The researchers found that people who took sleeping pills had four times the mortality rate of the group with no sleeping pill prescriptions. Even patients prescribed less than eighteen doses per year were more likely to die during the study period than those who did not take any sleeping pills. Equally as worrying is the finding that there was a 35% increase in the development of cancer in those who had been prescribed more than 132 doses per year.

Despite these potentially serious health outcomes some may still choose to pop a pill as it seems like an easy option. But I would encourage you to stop and ask yourself this question:

'If the sleeping pills are solving my sleep problem why do I continue to take them?'

The answer is blatantly clear. The sleeping pill does not solve the underlying issue of your sleeplessness: it merely allows for a chemically induced sleep, often leaving you feeling not so great the next day.

A better approach would be to speak with your doctor about the need to continue taking sleeping pills and to start investigating the underlying cause (or causes) of your sleeplessness. Armed with that information you can start implementing permanent solutions and look forward to the day (or night) when all you need as a sleeping aid is a comfortable bed and pillow.

Chapter 2

What is sleep?

BEFORE WE LEARN HOW TO achieve good sleep on a regular basis it is helpful to have a measure of what we are aiming for. When we have disturbed sleep almost every night, we begin to think that all the world, apart from ourselves, have deep, restful sleep night after night, year after year, awaking refreshed every morning and ready to greet the challenges of the day.

It is easy to be seduced into the idea of a TV bedding commercial where we commonly see people leaping out of bed, smiling and laughing after a most fantastic night of sleep. As with almost every other TV commercial though, the reality is far more prosaic. Even the best of sleepers will have nights when they do not sleep well, when they wake up wanting more sleep than they got, and then struggle with tiredness the following day.

It is important therefore that we set ourselves realistic expectations. Linda – a self-professed great sleeper – provides an excellent demonstration of what realistic expectations are.

Linda's story

Linda cannot remember a time she did not sleep well. When she talks about her sleep she explains that once she goes to bed, normally between 10 and 10.30 pm, she falls asleep within about 15 minutes and sleeps soundly, undisturbed, until she wakes the next morning at around 6.30 am. She says she keeps this routine regardless of what is happening in her life. Indeed the only thing that concerns her about her sleep is that she needs at least 8 hours (ideally 8 and a half hours) of sleep to function optimally.

This constantly undisturbed sleep may seem too good to be true – and it is. What Linda is actually recalling is her sleeping profile over recent months. When asked to recall any event in her life that had been traumatic she quickly remembered that her sleep at such a time had been 'truly dreadful'. Three years previously she had discovered that her husband was having an affair and her life had been turned upside down. Apart from everything else that was going wrong she remembered how desperately she yearned for a good night's sleep. At that time she would lie in bed awake for hours and when she finally managed to get to sleep it was fitful and not at all restful, leaving her feeling exhausted the next day. Her poor sleep had continued for quite some time – probably on and off for about 6 months.

As she talked about it she was surprised that she had completely forgotten her poor sleeping during this period of her life and it made her realise that perhaps she was not always the perfect sleeper. As she warmed to the topic she realised that there had been the odd night even in recent times when her sleep had been less than ideal. For example, when she'd started her new job, she had tossed and turned for a lot of the night. She also realised that sometimes her sleep was in fact disturbed by the need to go to the toilet in the early hours of the morning and occasionally it took her a little while to fall back to sleep. Linda's realisation that the perception of herself as a great sleeper was a little tarnished by a few nights of poor sleep is much closer to the reality for most of us.

It would be almost impossible to find someone who always, without fail, had great sleep. There will always be events in life that have the potential to disturb our sleep. This is not only completely normal but it is to be expected. The difference is that those people who generally sleep well, like Linda, tend to only remember the good sleep and have little memory of periods of poor sleep.

Sleeping well doesn't mean that once you overcome your current sleeping problem you will always, no matter what, have great sleep. Rather, understanding the processes of sleep and mastering them will help you achieve deep and restful sleep more often. When it comes to sleep all of us are individuals and have different requirements as to when we sleep and how much sleep we need. Some of us will need 7 hours and some will need 9 (and a very small minority, about 3%, will only need about 5–6 hours). Some will want to go to sleep at 8 pm and others at midnight.

Whatever our sleep profile, we need to understand it and make it work for us. Sometimes this may be difficult as many of us do not sleep alone, and it may be necessary to seek the aid of our partner to help us evaluate our sleep and make it work for us. Once we are able to do this though we too will have 'normal' sleep – although it may well look different to Linda's 'normal' sleep. Moreover as time goes on and good sleep becomes our norm, most of us will find that we too will become like Linda and think that almost nothing disturbs our sleep because we don't give sleep much thought at all.

Understanding sleep

An important first step in improving sleep is understanding what sleep is and how our body manages it. Even though we may not realise it, sleep is a complex process and understanding some of these complexities is critical to our quest for good, consolidated sleep on a regular basis.

So what is sleep? Surprising as it may seem, not all sleep is the same. We actually have two different types of sleep: Non-Rapid Eye Movement sleep (NREM sleep) and Rapid Eye Movement sleep

(REM sleep). Both types of sleep are essential to our ongoing mental and physical well-being.

NREM sleep has three stages. Stages 1 and 2 are often referred to as light sleep and stage 3 is more commonly known as deep sleep or slow wave sleep (SWS). When we go to sleep we initially go into light sleep. As we fall more asleep we descend into deep sleep. Depending on how tired we are we will be in deep sleep within 10–25 minutes of falling asleep – the more tired we are, the quicker we get into deep sleep.

Once in deep sleep, we will remain in that state for up to 40 minutes. This stage of sleep is quite different to light sleep. During the light stages of sleep we can be easily woken up, but in deep sleep we become difficult to arouse. If we are awakened from this stage of sleep we will generally feel disorientated and may have trouble functioning well. This feeling of grogginess has a name – sleep inertia. Depending on the circumstances, sleep inertia can last for several minutes and rarely exceeds 30 minutes, except in cases of major sleep deprivation where it may last much longer. Sleep inertia is commonly experienced upon waking in the morning after our night sleep, especially if we have had insufficient sleep, but it is felt more severely if we are aroused abruptly from deep sleep – as may occur after a long afternoon sleep. The difficulty in arousing from deep sleep is an important characteristic of stage 3 because it is in this sleep state that our body's repair and hormonal systems are active. This is why a consolidated deep sleep is essential for a healthy body and healthy metabolism.

After deep sleep the body goes into REM sleep. This sleep is often referred to as dream sleep. We are usually able to observe if someone is dreaming (especially babies) because there will be movements beneath their eyelids as well as eyelashes moving (these are the rapid eye movements that give the name to this sleep state). Dream sleep has some different characteristics to NREM sleep.

Although our brains are very active in dream sleep, our body is not, and it is during this sleep state that most of our muscles are paralysed – only our eye muscles and diaphragm (for breathing) maintain their ability to move. There is a very good reason why the majority of our muscles are paralysed when we dream. Most of us at some stage have experienced a dream where we were trying to run away from something only to find that all we could do was drag our hands and feet very, very slowly. The reason for this is that while dreaming we were in fact *trying* to move but luckily couldn't because our muscle paralysis was protecting us from acting out our dreams.

Something to note

While it is true that most adults (about 97%) require between 7–9 hours' sleep, there are some people who have a special 'short sleep' gene. This means that these people only require 5–6 hours of sleep per night. On the other hand, people with the 'long sleep' gene need 9–10 hours of sleep each night.

Sleep length is a genetic-specific characteristic so varying sleep needs tend to run in families. If your father or mother was a short (or long) sleeper then chances are you will be too. But it should be remembered that for the vast majority of adults there is a need for 7–9 hours of sleep every 24 hours.

In the same way that deep sleep is vital to our physical health, dream sleep is essential for our mental health and critically important to our ability to learn. Without sufficient dream sleep our ability to think and learn is severely impaired.

A normal sleep pattern is between 7–9 hours of consolidated sleep. In these hours we cycle through the sleep stages going from stage 1 NREM sleep to stage 2 NREM sleep to stage 3 NREM sleep through to REM sleep and then back to the start of the cycle. We continue to cycle like this throughout the night for the entire sleep period. The diagram on the next page tracks this cycling and, for anyone experiencing insomnia, this is an important diagram to understand because it explains why you may be vulnerable to night-time awakenings.

If we look at this diagram (also called a hypnogram) we can see that:

- Each sleep cycle takes about 90 minutes, with more deep sleep in the first half of the night and more REM sleep (or dream sleep) in the second half.

- Once we decide to go to sleep and turn out the light we will spend some time in wakefulness. The time it takes to fall asleep is called sleep latency and is often used as an indicator of how tired we are. For example, falling asleep within 5 minutes of lights out (5-minute sleep latency) is indicative of severe tiredness.
- If we are not sleep deprived our sleep latency will be anywhere between 10–20 minutes. Sometimes people with insomnia have trouble with this part of their sleep and their sleep latency may be as great as 1.5–2 hours. (This type of insomnia is referred to as sleep-onset insomnia and will be discussed over the next few chapters).
- Once asleep it will take about 15–25 minutes to get into deep sleep (depending on how tired we are). In the first cycle of the night we will remain in deep sleep for about the next 40 minutes.
- After this time we will start our dream sleep. In this first cycle of the night we only spend a brief amount of time in dream sleep and following this we start the cycle again.

A normal sleep pattern

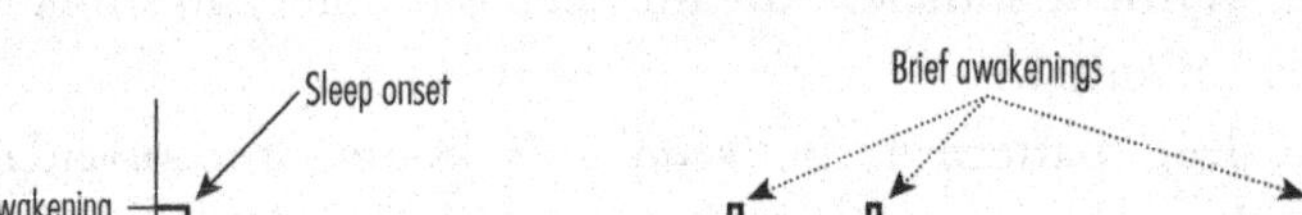

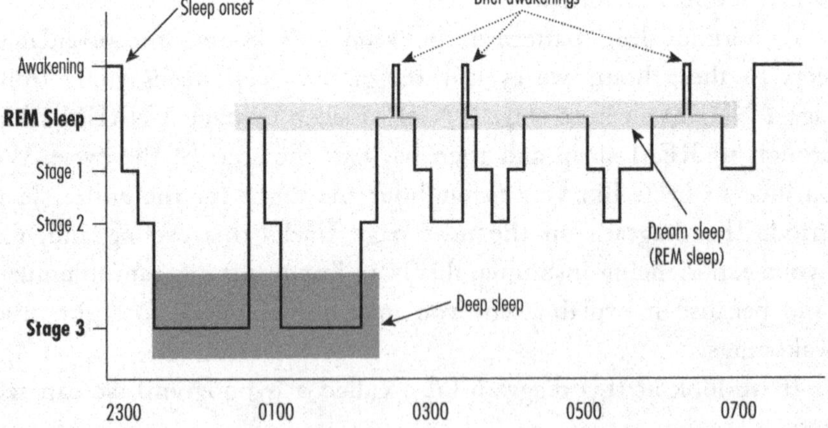

The movement through the various sleep cycles is an important process to understand because when we transit through them we often, but not always, experience a brief wakeful period. Most of us have no recollection of these brief wakeful periods but for many of us who struggle with sleep, these times of transit are when we are particularly vulnerable to being woken up.

Myth busting

A recent theory has suggested that because our sleep cycles are 90 minutes long we should sleep for multiples of 90 minutes. In other words, we should sleep for either 7.5 hours or 9 hours. This is not true.

Firstly, the length of our sleep cycle is varied and is between 90–110 minutes. Secondly, there is no consequence to awakening from any particular sleep stage (although if we wake from deep sleep we are more likely to experience sleep inertia). What is true, however, is that we are much more easily woken up from light sleep or dream sleep than from deep sleep.

Generally, because most of us are tired when we go to sleep at night, it is usual that we get at least one full cycle of sleep, and, more often than not, two full sleep cycles (around 180 minutes), without much disturbance. Those who struggle to maintain sleep will frequently find they will wake up around 3 hours after they go to sleep – roughly the time it takes to go through two full sleep cycles and approximately the same time as they transit through dream sleep to light sleep.

As we have learned, we are easily aroused from light sleep, and if we have fragile sleep it means that at these times we will often fully wake up and find it difficult to return to sleep. Once we do manage to get back to sleep, the next time we go through light sleep (about 1.5 hours later) we may again experience another episode of wakefulness, and so it can go on throughout the night leading to what feels like a largely sleepless night. This type of sleeplessness is referred to as sleep-maintenance insomnia and will be discussed over the next few chapters.

For now though it is important to remember what we have just learned: sleep is not a unitary state. Sleeping involves cycling through all the sleep states – Stages 1, 2 and 3 NREM sleep and REM sleep – as well as having brief periods of wakefulness. Each of these sleep states have particular characteristics that are vitally important to our health and well-being: our NREM sleep is essential for a rested and repaired body and for a healthy metabolism and our REM sleep is critical to how well we think and feel.

By recognising the various stages of sleep and understanding how we cycle through them during our sleep period we can begin to break down the mystery of sleep. Also, because we now know that we are more easily awoken from some sleep states (stages 1 and 2 NREM and REM sleep) than from others (stage 3 NREM or deep sleep) we can appreciate why we wake up more easily at particular times of the night than at other times.

Keeping all this in mind, we are now ready to learn some more about the sleep process.

Chapter 3

The process of sleep

FOR MOST OF US, OUR sleep pattern has a particular regularity, which is one of the more important features of sleep – sleep is not a random activity. People the world over, regardless of culture, tend to fall asleep, or want to fall asleep, somewhere between 9 pm and midnight and wake up the next day somewhere between 6 am and 9 am. This pattern of sleep has existed for millennia and made good sense in the days of cave-dwellers, where it was dangerous to be out and about in the dark. Even though we now have the ability, due to electric lighting, to be awake (or asleep) and productive any time during our 24-hour day we continue to retain this pattern of sleeping during the dark hours. Of course some in our society, such as those who work shifts, do not sleep according to this pattern and are productive in the night hours. But the majority of shift-workers will agree, the sleep they want the most and the sleep they find the best is the overnight sleep. This universality of sleep-timing suggests that sleeping in the night hours is a biological necessity – which indeed it is.

The persistence of this consistent sleeping pattern is due to the fact that our ability to sleep is a finely modulated process that balances two different needs: the necessity of getting the right amount of sleep

(7–9 hours), and the necessity for this to occur during the dark hours. In order to achieve the appropriate balance the body links both our need for sleep (or sleep drive) with our in-built biological 24-hour cycle of sleep/wakefulness, and it is due to this linking that we are able to have a consolidated overnight sleep period.

Sleep drive

Simply put, our sleep drive is our need for sleep. Provided we get the amount of sleep that we require, our sleep drive is at a minimum when we wake up. As the day progresses and the amount of time since we got out of bed in the morning increases the more tired we become, and hence our sleep drive (or need for sleep) increases.

Our increasing sleep drive is a consequence of the build-up of a chemical in our brain called adenosine. This is the chemical that makes us feel sleepy. As soon as we wake up in the morning our brain starts to produce adenosine and continues to produce it while we are awake. As soon as we go to sleep though, the brain stops producing it and the level of this sleep-inducing chemical rapidly drops away. If we get sufficient sleep, the level of adenosine in our brain is minimal when we wake up the next day so we feel refreshed and vitalised and, most importantly, we no longer feel sleepy. If we do not get enough sleep, however, the level of adenosine will still be high the next morning and we'll find it difficult to wake up and will probably feel particularly sleepy at certain times during the day.

Something to think about

Have you ever wondered why coffee is so effective at giving a short burst of alertness? It turns out the longer we are awake the more sleepy chemicals our brain produces. In particular, adenosine builds up in our brain and this sleepy chemical determines how tired we feel. When we have caffeine it successfully masks the effects of adenosine so it cannot do its job. In a way caffeine fools the brain into thinking there is very little of the sleepy chemical. This is great in the short term, because it makes us feel less sleepy, but when the effects of caffeine wear off all the adenosine that has been produced in the interim is unmasked and you can suddenly succumb to an overwhelming sleep urge (as in the case of a sleepy driver).

Circadian rhythm of alertness

Our 24-hour biological cycles are also known as our internal 24-hour body clock or our circadian rhythms (from the Latin *circa*, meaning approximately, and *dies*, meaning day). Regardless of what we call them these cycles control many of our bodily functions – when we get hungry, when we go to the toilet, when we produce certain hormones, our highs and lows of blood pressure and body temperature, when we feel most alert, when we have the greatest co-ordination and so on. Importantly though, our circadian rhythms play a critical role in sleep and the rhythm most central to sleep is our 24-hour cycle of alertness.

Our body has an alternating cycle of sleepy and alert periods throughout the 24-hour day. We have two periods in the day when we feel most awake and two periods when we feel most sleepy. This cycle of alert and non-alert periods is illustrated in the diagram below.

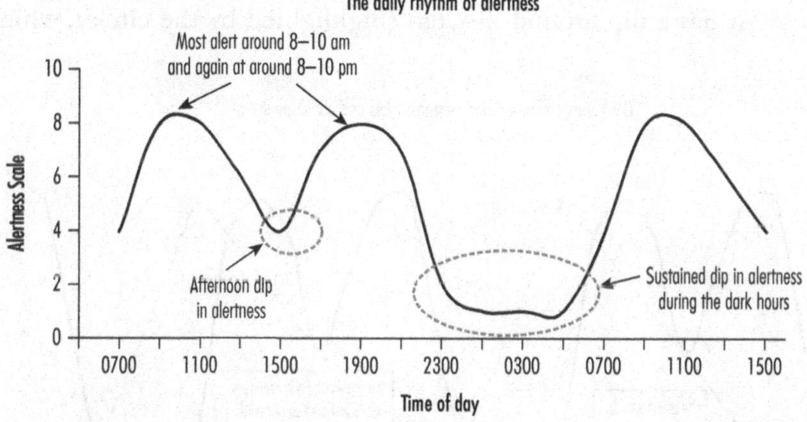

We can see in this diagram that there is a wave pattern with two periods of increased alertness, one around 8–10 am and then again at 8–10 pm; and two periods of minimum alertness, around 2–4 pm and again at around 1–5 am. The periods of minimal alertness are marked by the circles.

The idea of different periods of alertness during the day comes as no surprise to most people. Many of us have experienced lethargy at mid-afternoon when we often reach for a caffeinated drink or a sweet snack to revive ourselves. Numerous cultures have respected this lull in alertness during the early afternoon hours – hence the idea of siestas.

By considering these two processes – our sleep drive and our cycle of alertness – together, we begin to see how there is a harmony between sleep drive and the cycle of alertness in the well-slept person, which allows them to fall asleep at a regular time and to sustain sleep for a regular and consolidated period.

This harmony is depicted in the diagram below that tracks these two processes over a 2-day period in a person who gets the right amount of sleep most nights.

Looking at this diagram we can see two lines. The dotted line is the sleep drive. In the morning at around 9.30 am the sleep drive is low. It rises throughout the day (due to the production of our sleepy chemical adenosine) until about 10.30 pm when the person goes to sleep. Over the sleep period (the shaded area), this person's sleep drive decreases to a minimum (as the level of adenosine decreases), at which point they wake up – around 7 am.

The solid line represents the 24-hour cycle of alertness. As we can see it has a dip around 2–4 pm (highlighted by the circle), which

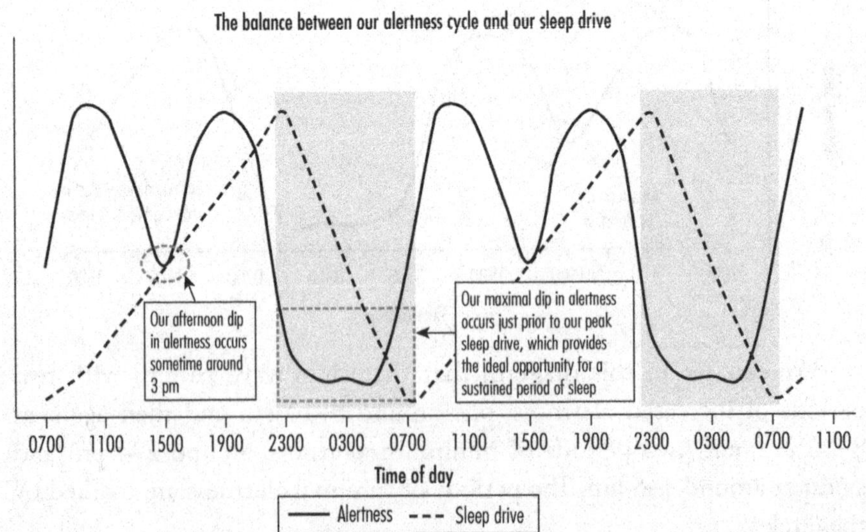

coincides with the afternoon sleepy period, and another substantial and sustained dip between about 10.30 pm and 6 am (dotted rectangle). This second dip in alertness coincides not just with the hours of darkness, but also occurs just prior to the maximum sleep drive – at which point sleep will happen (shaded area).

It is not just coincidence that the 6-hour dip in alertness begins just before our maximum sleep drive – nature intended it that way. By ensuring that we are beginning our minimal alertness period around the same time as we have the greatest sleep drive, we are able to obtain the consolidated sleep so essential to our health and well-being. However, when we disrupt this harmony, getting to sleep or staying asleep can become very difficult. It is at these times many of us are surprised that even though we feel extremely tired when we go to bed, we either cannot get to sleep or we find it difficult to maintain sleep.

For most of us this happens only occasionally, but for those of us with insomnia it happens on a frequent basis and is very distressing. Although the level of distress is considerably different when we compare an occasional bad night of sleep to almost nightly sleeplessness, the disruption in the sleep process itself may be substantially the same. We can understand this similarity a little more if we consider John's attempts at getting to sleep early one night.

John's story

John had not slept much the night before and had been feeling tired all day. He decided that instead of going to bed at his normal time (10.30 pm) he would go to bed at 8 pm. Even though he was feeling very tired (and had a high sleep drive), he could not get to sleep, and he ended up getting out of bed about 20 minutes later, feeling quite awake. While John was annoyed, he could have predicted this if he had understood the sleep process. John had been trying to sleep when his body was feeling the most alert and so naturally sleep was elusive. Far better if John had:

1. Recognised his peak alertness occurred around 9 pm and went to bed *after* that time rather than before it. In this way John would

have been working in synchrony with his circadian rhythm of alertness *and* his sleep drive. He would have therefore fallen asleep quickly due to his increased sleep drive, even though it was earlier than his normal bedtime.

2. Alternatively, John could have alleviated his tiredness by recognising that there is a time during the day when his sleep drive and his cycle of alertness work together, which would allow him to sleep a little in order to decrease his feelings of sleepiness. If John was at home, he should have tried to nap in the afternoon hours (around 3 pm) when his alertness cycle was at a low. If he had done this, for just 20 minutes, he would have successfully decreased the amount of sleepy chemicals in his brain, allowing him to feel more energetic and awake until it was time to go to bed that night (*after* his alertness peak). This is the idea behind the power nap. Care must always be taken, however, to ensure the nap goes no longer than 20 minutes (a timer or alarm may need to be used) as otherwise getting to sleep that night may be difficult.

The Power Nap

If we are feeling tired and not very productive it may be a good idea to take a 20-minute power nap. By napping for no more than this amount of time we ensure that we stay only in the light stages of sleep (stages 1 and 2 NREM). If we sleep any longer we may go into deep sleep and we will then find it very difficult to wake up. We may also experience prolonged sleep inertia, which will make us feel even more tired and dazed than before we took our nap. The secret, therefore, is to restrict the nap to 20 minutes, which is sufficient time to decrease our feelings of sleepiness while also allowing us to wake up feeling more refreshed and energised.

Understanding the interconnectedness of sleep drive and the cycle of alertness is critical if we are going to improve our sleep. It is especially important that each of us understands our own pattern because, while peak alertness occurs around 9 pm for the majority of us, for some, peak alertness may occur as early as 7 pm or as late as 1 am. In order for us to get the best night's sleep possible it is essential to know when we experience our peak alertness, because it is this that largely determines when we *can* get to sleep.

Many of us are already aware whether we are a lark (early to bed and to wake) or an owl (late to bed and late to wake), but few people really know when they have their evening peak in alertness or their afternoon lull.

Owls and larks

Larks like to go to bed early and get up early. They enjoy the morning and are often at their most productive at this time. Owls, on the other hand, are not morning people and frequently struggle to get out of bed. They much prefer the evening hours and may do some of their best work at this time.

While there are some people who seem to be quite judgemental about owls – believing that they are lazier and less productive than larks – there is no research to show that either type has any advantage over, or works harder than, the other. The only true difference between the lark and the owl is the slightly different times that they experience their peak alert and sleepy times. If this is understood, and not considered as either a positive or a negative trait, both larks and owls can use their knowledge of their individual pattern of alertness to maximise their productivity.

The evening peak in alertness is important because, unless we have a very high sleep drive, if we try to go to sleep before this we will not be able to get to sleep, resulting in a long sleep latency (time it takes to get to sleep). Knowing when our afternoon lull occurs is also important because we can minimise activities that require vigilance at that time, such as driving a long distance.

There is an easy way to find out our personal cycle of alertness. By tracking how we feel throughout the day we will quickly be able to see when we are at our most alert and when we are feeling the most non-alert.

What is your cycle of alertness?

To discover your alertness cycle read through the example 'Determining Susan's cycle of alertness' and, using that as your guide, fill in the table below using the same scale. Do this over a 4-day period.

	0700	0900	1100	1300	1500	1700	1900	2100	2300	0100	0300	0500
Day 1												
Day 2												
Day 3												
Day 4												

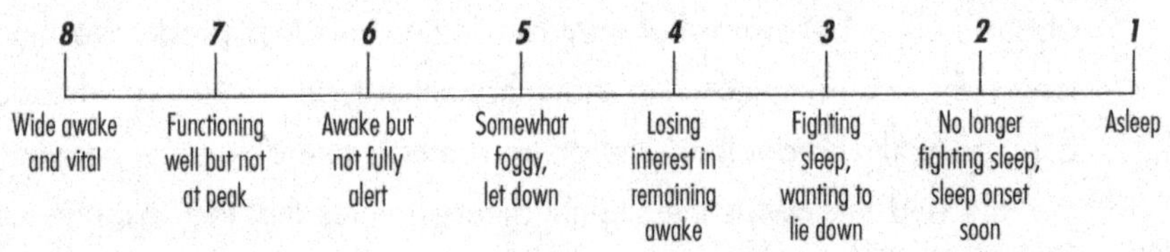

Adapted from the Stanford Sleepiness Scale

Determining Susan's cycle of alertness

Susan was studying for her final exams and wanted to optimise her studying time. She was aware that there were times of the day when she was able to be most productive but she was not absolutely sure when those times were. As a result she sometimes made the mistake of not making the most of these times. To ensure that she appropriately planned her study times so that they coincided with her most alert periods Susan followed her feelings of alertness throughout the day and recorded them in the table below.

At 7 am (0700) Susan felt awake but not fully alert, so she gave herself a 6 in the 0700 column. By 0900 she felt wide awake and recorded an 8 in the 0900 column. She still felt wide awake at 1100 so recorded another 8. At 1300 Susan was no longer feeling fully alert and gave herself a 6. At 1500 she felt tired and unmotivated, so she recorded a 4. At 1700 she's functioning well, but not at peak so recorded a 7. She felt great and wide awake at 1900 and therefore recorded an 8. At 2100 she's no longer at her peak, so recorded a 7; at 2300 she's just about to fall off to sleep so recorded a 2. She was asleep at 0100, 0300 and 0500 so records a 1 in those columns.

Once Susan saw the results of her alertness tracking she quickly worked out that her best study times were between about 8 am and 1 pm, and between about 5 pm and 9 pm, with possibly a power nap around 3 pm. She also was able to work out that the best time to stop working in the evening was around 9.30 pm as her alertness was decreasing and she was far better off at this point putting her books away and starting to prepare her body for sleep.

	0700	0900	1100	1300	1500	1700	1900	2100	2300	0100	0300	0500
Day 1	6	8	8	6	4	7	8	7	2	1	1	1

By doing this exercise we can quickly determine, as did Susan, our individual cycle of alertness and use this knowledge to perform our more difficult tasks when we are most alert and to plan our bedtime when we are most likely to fall asleep.

Owl or extreme owl?

What will become apparent from doing this exercise is whether our personal circadian rhythm of alertness is similar to the majority of people, whose evening peak occurs around 8–9 pm, or whether it is considerably earlier or later than this peak. If we find that our peak evening alertness actually happens around 11 pm (or even later) this tells us that we are definitely an owl and, depending on exactly how late our peak of alertness occurs, we may be an 'extreme owl'.

If this is you, it may mean that you have spent a lot of time trying to go to sleep before your internal peak but, because your alertness is high, you regularly lie in bed trying to get to sleep for a long time without much success. Sometimes you will fall asleep quickly. If we were to plot your sleep drive though, the times you fall asleep easily would probably coincide with times that your sleep drive was really high. In these cases sleep onset isn't a harmony of the processes, but due only to the overriding sleep drive that you are experiencing. When sleep is only the consequence of a high sleep drive, sleep onset may be rapid but the sleeping period may be short-lived, especially if we fall asleep one or two hours before the peak in our alertness.

Lark or extreme lark?

In a similar, but opposite way, it may be that after doing the alertness cycle we find that our evening peak occurs as early as 7 pm and our morning peak occurs, not at 9 am, but rather somewhere around 6–7 am. If this is you this indicates that you are a lark and, depending on just how early your morning peak of alertness is, you could be an 'extreme lark'. In the same way that the extreme owl will lie awake at night trying to get to sleep, the extreme lark will wake up very early in the morning and be unable to return to sleep. In many cases, this can lead to early-morning awakening insomnia.

If you are an extreme lark or an extreme owl, don't despair. There are ways of manipulating your circadian rhythm of alertness so that you can get to sleep at a reasonable time and stay asleep for a consolidated period. To determine whether you are an extreme owl or lark it is necessary to know your cycle of alertness, so do take the time over the next few days to map out your cycle.

What sets the circadian rhythm?

In later chapters, we will talk in more detail about how to manipulate your alertness levels so that they work for you rather than against you, but first let's learn more about how they are determined and exactly how our 24-hour body clock is set.

Apart from the daily cycle evident in our sleeping pattern, circadian rhythms are also evident in our appetite patterns, body temperature cycle, hormone production, gastrointestinal regulation, cardiovascular regulation and countless other bodily processes. These cycles are created internally in the brain in what is commonly referred to as our body clock (scientifically known as the Suprachiasmatic Nucleus, or the SCN). The primary determiner of these rhythms is sunlight.

How this is achieved is quite simple. Sunlight enters our brain through our eyes (the optic nerve) and is registered by the SCN. Once the SCN has registered the light, it will switch on (or switch off) the various hormonal systems that are needed to regulate the daily rhythms mentioned earlier, and it will do this at appropriate times during the day or night. Understanding just some of the various circadian rhythms will give us an insight into how to ensure deep, restful sleep.

The vampire hormone – melatonin

Melatonin is sometimes referred to as the hormone of darkness or the 'vampire' hormone because it is secreted only when light begins to fade, then increases in concentration during the night hours, decreases as soon as it detects light and is almost non-existent in our bodies during the sunlight hours. Melatonin is produced in the brain and once fading light is detected the melatonin level in the blood begins to rise (normally at around 8–9 pm). It remains high for the next 8–10 hours, until the sun starts to rise at which time the melatonin level begins to decrease such that by about 8–9 am it is back to its minimal daytime level.

Melatonin is critical to the setting of our 24-hour body clock and the timing of our circadian rhythms. In fact it is so fundamental that it can be thought of as the master of our biological clock. If bright lighting (including computer screens, TVs and smart phones) prevents our SCN from detecting fading light and the secretion of melatonin is delayed, there will be a delay in all our 24-hour cycles, including the cycle of alertness, and we will have difficulty falling asleep.

On the other hand, if the SCN has detected fading light earlier than normal, melatonin secretion will start earlier and consequently other body cycles will also begin earlier. Many of us may have experienced this unknowingly in the past when we have been camping. It is common to feel more tired and go to sleep earlier than usual when camping and we may think that this is due to the fresh air and great outdoors we are experiencing – but this is not the only reason. When we go camping our exposure to artificial light is very limited and as a result our eye detects the fading light as soon as the sun goes down and hence the earlier secretion of melatonin, and the earlier bedtime.

The timing of melatonin secretion is critical to our ability to go to sleep. When we start to produce melatonin it signals to the body that it is dark and time to prepare for sleep. As a result, about an hour after melatonin levels start to rise, our alertness starts to decline and we begin to feel sleepy, and if we are in a position to fall asleep we will be able to do so. Not only is melatonin important in assisting us in getting to sleep, it is also important in maintaining sleep. If for some reason our melatonin levels start to decrease during the night (for example, a bright light comes into the room) we will be less likely to maintain sleep.

The body is marvellous and the harmony of the secretion of melatonin upon fading light combined with the decline in our alertness creates a perfect environment for consolidated sleep. Unfortunately, modern man has unknowingly upset this harmony, and for many of us the perfect environment for sleep has become elusive.

Light and vampires don't mix

Over 100 years ago the electric light bulb was invented. While this was a wonderful invention and we would be lost without it, it has come at a cost. Most of us now have access to artificial light 24 hours a day, every day of the year, which means the night hours need no longer be characterised by fading light and this change has had a significant effect on the biological sleep process.

For many of us it turns out that what was a wonderful leap for industry and productivity was not such a great leap forward for our physiology. While the body can adapt well, it has not yet learned to differentiate between sunlight and artificial light. This means when we are exposed to artificial light rather than fading light our brains won't start melatonin secretion. Without this we will not begin to feel the necessary sleepiness that tells our body it is time to go to sleep and this can cause difficulties in either getting to sleep or maintaining sleep.

The 24-hour temperature cycle

Melatonin not only sets our alertness cycle but it is also responsible for setting other 24-hour cycles, especially those that are involved in sleep – the two primary ones being the circadian rhythm of alertness (already discussed) and the circadian rhythm of our temperature cycle.

While we may not be aware of it, our core body temperature fluctuates throughout the day. It does not fluctuate by much – there is only one degree of difference between our usual minimum (36°C) and maximum (37°C) temperatures – but, despite this, our core body temperature greatly affects our ability to initiate sleep and to stay asleep. The rhythm of our temperature cycle is shown in the diagram below.

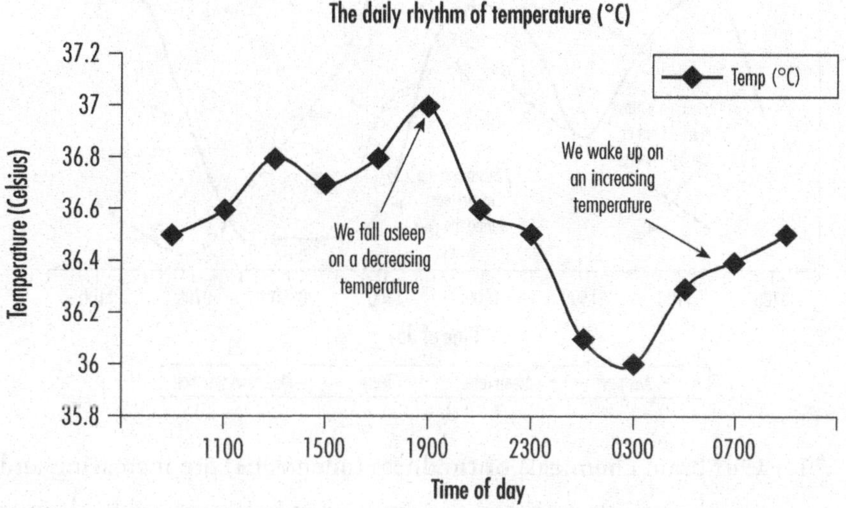

In this diagram we can see that we have a maximum body temperature at about 7 pm and a minimum body temperature at about 4 am. Even though the fluctuation of temperature is not great, we normally find it easier to fall asleep on a decreasing temperature (after 7 pm) and awake on an increasing temperature (after 4 am). If we disrupt this cycle, we may find it difficult to either get to sleep or stay asleep.

Putting it all together

If we think about the cycles we have talked about, and look at the diagrams again, we will realise there is a happy coincidence. To show just how marvellously our body works I have combined the circadian rhythms of alertness and temperature with the 24-hour light/dark cycle of melatonin secretion in the one diagram and placed them in the context of the increasing sleep drive that we experience as the day goes on.

In this diagram, four things are happening simultaneously between the hours of 7 pm and 10 pm that are preparing us for sleep:

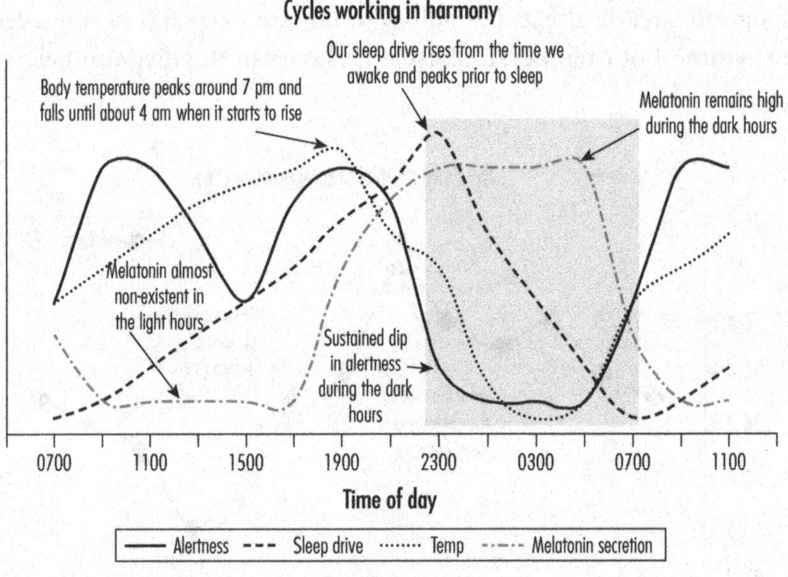

1. Our brain chemicals of tiredness (adenosine) are increasing and our sleep drive reaches a maximum just before we go to sleep at around 10.30 pm (black dashed line).
2. The light begins to fade, the SCN detects this and our brain begins to secrete our sleep hormone, melatonin (grey dash-dotted line).
3. Our body temperature begins to decrease, preparing us for sleeping (grey dotted line).

4. Our cycle of alertness is decreasing and over the next 6 hours we will experience a low in this circadian rhythm (black solid line).

The fact that all four things occur within such a small timeframe means that each night there is an ideal time for us to fall asleep and to maintain sleep (indicated by the grey shaded area). It is the synchrony of these rhythms that enables us to sleep long and well.

If we create a disturbance in this harmonious process we will have problems: we may not be able to get to sleep, we may not be able to get enough sleep, or we may not be able to maintain our sleep. For however long the disruptions are maintained we will have problems with sleep.

Sometimes the disruption will only be for a short period of time, but all too often these brief periods of sleeplessness turn into the long-term problem of chronic sleeplessness with all its accompanying health, mood and behavioural problems.

However, the good news is that we are now well on the path to overcoming our sleeplessness issues, because our new-found understanding of what sleep is and how it occurs is the first step in the process of unravelling our individual sleeping difficulties.

Chapter 4

Insomnia

OVER THE NEXT FEW CHAPTERS we are going to examine how our sleep processes intersect with the various types of insomnia, learn what science can tell us about this and hopefully discover just what it is that is causing your specific sleep problem.

While there are a number of possible starting points for this investigation we will begin with the problem of chronic insomnia – partly because of the seriousness of the condition, but also because if we master chronic insomnia, we have just about mastered most aspects of sleep.

So what is chronic insomnia? Medically speaking, a person will be considered to have chronic insomnia when they have been having inadequate sleep 3 or more nights per week over a period of more than 6 months, and this has caused them to feel all the consequences of poor sleep that we talked about previously – tiredness, exhaustion, irritability, difficulty concentrating, problems with learning and so on.

When assessing and treating chronic insomnia it is always worthwhile evaluating just how badly sleeplessness is affecting you at the beginning of treatment. This is because we often forget how awful we may have felt at the start and so we sometimes don't notice small improvements. By filling in the table below you will be able to score the severity of your insomnia as it is affecting you right now, and then as you implement strategies to improve your sleep you can re-do the assessment. This will help you evaluate how effective the interventions that you implement are.

When you have completed the table make sure to keep a record of the score and the date because as you go through the book and start improving your sleep you will be able to see objectively just how far you have come in your quest to improve your sleep.

	Assessing the severity of insomnia					
	0	1	2	3	4	Score
Indicate the severity of your sleep problem: * Difficulty falling asleep * Difficulty staying asleep * Problems waking up too early	 None None None	 Mild Mild Mild	 Moderate Moderate Moderate	 Severe Severe Severe	 Very severe Very severe Very severe	
How satisfied/dissatisfied are you with your current sleep pattern?	Very satisfied	Satisfied	Moderately satisfied	Dissatisfied	Very dissatisfied	
How noticeable to others do you think your sleep problem is in terms of impairing your quality of life?	Not at all noticeable	A little	Somewhat	Much	Very much noticeable	
How worried/distressed are you about your current sleep problem?	Not at all worried	A little	Somewhat	Much	Very much worried	
To what extent do you consider your current sleep problem to interfere with your daily functioning (e.g. daytime fatigue, mood, ability to function at work/school/daily chores, concentration, memory, mood)?	Not interfering	A little	Somewhat	Much	Very much interfering	

Total Score: Add up the number of points for each.

Interpretation: *0–7 = no significant insomnia; 8–14 = sub-threshold insomnia; 15–21 = clinical insomnia (moderate severity); 22–28 = clinical insomnia (severe).*

Types of sleeplessness

Once you have an idea of the current severity of your sleep problem we can start to learn more about how we can systematically deal with the complexities of sleeplessness. There is more than one type of chronic poor sleep and the different types are generally categorised by the time at which the sleep problem occurs.

It may be that we have difficulty falling asleep and lie in bed for hours trying to get to sleep to no avail. This type of insomnia is often referred to as a sleep-onset or sleep-initiation insomnia.

On the other hand it may be that we have absolutely no problem with going to sleep but have considerable problems staying asleep. We might often find ourselves awake 1 hour after going to sleep, and then again 2 hours after going back to sleep and so on throughout the night. This type of insomnia is referred to as sleep-maintenance insomnia.

Finally, it may be that we get to sleep easily, stay asleep easily but wake in the early morning hours and lie awake, unable to go back to sleep, until the sun comes up. This is known as early-morning-awakening insomnia.

Of course, just because sleep troubles are categorised in this rather simplistic manner does not mean that we cannot have any combination of the above. It may be that we have both sleep-onset and sleep-maintenance insomnia, or both sleep-onset and early-morning-awakening insomnia. In situations like these we will need to understand what causes each type of insomnia and how each can be treated.

The initial step, in any treatment for sleeplessness, is to label the problem according to the above categorisation. An easy way to manage this is to complete the sleep diary at the end of this chapter. After filling in the diary for one week it will become clear what type of insomnia you have, your average sleep time and how many times a week you have difficulty sleeping.

It may be that you already have a good idea of your type of insomnia but, as before, it is important firstly to confirm this and secondly to record this information at the beginning of treatment so any improvement is easily seen. For example, if at the moment you are waking at 3 am unable to get back to sleep and in 2 weeks' time you are waking at 5 am unable to get back to sleep, even though you still won't be exactly where you want to be, you will be able to see a definite improvement and feel encouraged and motivated to continue with the process of improving your sleep.

Once you have worked out the category (or categories) of your sleep problem, the next thing is to work out whether the sleeplessness you are experiencing is secondary or primary.

Secondary insomnia

Secondary insomnia means that the sleeplessness you are experiencing is actually caused by another problem. With secondary insomnia we need to firstly determine the problem causing the sleeplessness and then to treat it. To understand this distinction a bit more let's look at Ted, who had a bad back. Ted had always slept well, but for the last 12 months he had been waking several times a night, finding it difficult to fall back asleep. As a result Ted was chronically sleep deprived and feeling exhausted most of the time, which only served to exacerbate his back pain. In an attempt to improve his pain Ted had back surgery and within weeks of the surgery he was mostly pain free. What made the surgery even more successful was that Ted began sleeping through the night again. Clearly Ted's sleeplessness was caused by his back pain, and once the pain was treated so too was the sleeplessness. In other words, Ted's insomnia was secondary to the back pain.

There are many and varied causes of secondary insomnia, which we will explore over the coming chapters. The good news is that secondary insomnia is often easier to treat than primary insomnia because by discovering the problem that is causing the sleeplessness and treating that, the insomnia will improve.

Primary insomnia

When insomnia is primary in nature it means there is no underlying problem that is causing the sleeplessness – it is a problem with the sleep process itself. To treat primary insomnia we need to examine the sleeping process. Primary insomnia may sometimes begin in childhood and the person suffering from it may not be able to remember a time when they ever slept well. More often though, primary chronic insomnia is a result of learned behaviour and sometimes people can vaguely trace it back to a point in time when they first started having problems with their sleep. Some of these possible points in time may include the onset of adolescence, starting work for the first time, the break-up of a marriage or death of a loved one.

Often though, people with primary insomnia are not aware of any trigger for their sleeplessness, they just know that it has been a long time since they had a good night's sleep.

If you suffer from primary insomnia, don't worry – it doesn't matter if you can remember a trigger or not. It is possible to resolve primary insomnia by implementing a range of practices which will be discussed later.

Common causes of sleeplessness

It is relatively common for people suffering from sleeplessness to self-diagnose primary insomnia and to leap to the conclusion that their insomnia is related to the way they approach sleep – they have had too much coffee, slept during the day or worked too late into the night. They are convinced that if only they can improve their sleep habits their sleep difficulties will resolve.

Don't get me wrong. Good sleep practices are absolutely critical for sound, refreshing sleep, but almost 90% of people suffer sleeplessness due to another problem, so all the best sleep practices in the world will not give us the sleep we crave if we have secondary insomnia.

So before a diagnosis of primary insomnia is made, it is absolutely imperative to rule out secondary insomnia. This is done by eliminating any other cause, such as a medical condition, psychological reason, sleep disorder or substance abuse.

In 2012 a research article was published which evaluated the causes of insomnia. The researchers discovered that primary insomnia was only one part of a much larger problem. In the sample group of nearly 1000 people, about 400 people reported difficulties sleeping but only 50 of them had primary insomnia; the rest had sleep difficulties due to another, underlying problem. The most common of these problems were:

- depression
- anxiety
- sleep apnoea
- another undiagnosed sleep disorder
- alcohol/substance abuse.

We will discuss each one of the secondary causes of insomnia revealed in the article later in the book and explore how we can find out whether or not this is your particular problem. We will also discuss strategies to overcome each problem.

Some of you will have none of these problems and your issue will indeed be primary insomnia, which we will also be discussing later. It's important though to read through the other sections and make sure you don't have another underlying secondary cause. Too many people assume they have primary insomnia and skip the secondary issues, and as a consequence continue to have poor sleep.

During this chapter we have spent a lot of time defining and talking about the various types of sleeplessness. Understanding the 'labels' is important because they help us isolate the particular issue causing the sleeplessness. If we do not understand the type of insomnia it will be more difficult to treat. It is important, therefore, to take the time to complete the sleep diary for a minimum of a week. Ideally you should try to continue with this until you are happy with how you sleep and thereafter to use it again if your sleep begins to be troublesome.

SLEEP DIARY WEEK 1

	I went to bed last night at:	I got out of bed this morning at:	Last night I was in bed for a total of:	Last night I fell asleep in about:	I woke up during the night:	During the night I was awake for a total of:	My sleep was disturbed by:	Last night I slept for a total of:	When I woke up for the day, I felt:	1 hour before going to sleep, I did . . .
Day Date	___ am/pm	___ am/pm	___ hours	___ minutes	___ # times	___ minutes		___ hours	Refreshed Somewhat refreshed Tired Very tired	
Day Date	___ am/pm	___ am/pm	___ hours	___ minutes	___ # times	___ minutes		___ hours	Refreshed Somewhat refreshed Tired Very tired	
Day Date	___ am/pm	___ am/pm	___ hours	___ minutes	___ # times	___ minutes		___ hours	Refreshed Somewhat refreshed Tired Very tired	
Day Date	___ am/pm	___ am/pm	___ hours	___ minutes	___ # times	___ minutes		___ hours	Refreshed Somewhat refreshed Tired Very tired	
Day Date	___ am/pm	___ am/pm	___ hours	___ minutes	___ # times	___ minutes		___ hours	Refreshed Somewhat refreshed Tired Very tired	
Day Date	___ am/pm	___ am/pm	___ hours	___ minutes	___ # times	___ minutes		___ hours	Refreshed Somewhat refreshed Tired Very tired	
Day Date	___ am/pm	___ am/pm	___ hours	___ minutes	___ # times	___ minutes		___ hours	Refreshed Somewhat refreshed Tired Very tired	

Chapter 5

Anxiety: is it keeping me awake?

BEFORE YOU TURN THE PAGE and decide this is not a chapter that applies to you, take the time to consider this fact: nearly 50% of people who struggle to have a good night's sleep also have anxiety.

This doesn't mean that half of the sleepless population is going around wringing their hands in a constantly worried state never knowing a moment of peace. Anxiety has become a dirty word, but all it really means is that some people are worried.

It seems to me that no one wants to be thought of as having 'anxiety' these days. But this has not always been the case and not so very long ago to say someone was 'anxious' was almost the same as saying someone was 'worried'.

In the 1980s the term Generalised Anxiety Disorder (GAD) was coined to describe intense and exaggerated worry which pervades everyday behaviour and which causes people to feel as if they were in imminent danger of some catastrophe.

The recognition of this disorder enabled access to therapies for the people who were experiencing it, but labelling the disorder as Generalised Anxiety Disorder resulted in a general perception that anxiety is an abnormal state of being and implied there's something wrong with being anxious. This causes many of us to go into denial when we are worried or concerned about anything. As a result it is often surprising for us to hear that worry/anxiety may be causing our sleep difficulties.

It is time to deal with the negative connotations surrounding the word anxiety and recognise that it is merely another form of worry.

Worried or anxious thoughts can stop us from getting to sleep at night. They can cause multiple awakenings during the night and they can even prevent us from going back to sleep when we wake up too early in the morning.

Anne's story

Anne was 45 years old, happily in a relationship, with two teenage children and a career that she loved. On the surface all was going well for her, except for one thing. She was experiencing the most terrible problems with her sleep. As a result she was feeling extremely tired all the time and often had an unreasonable irritability towards even the most minor of problems. In the last month or so she had begun to realise that her tiredness was also having a negative impact on her relationship with her husband.

In the past Anne had occasionally experienced bouts of insomnia and had taken sleeping pills. On these occasions, her difficulty sleeping seemed to eventually resolve and she would return to a normal sleeping pattern.

Over the years Anne had read a few books on how to get a good night's sleep and when I met her had developed a good going-to-bed routine which normally would have worked well. Her good night-time practices were not working very well for her anymore though. Her latest episode of insomnia had been going on for at least a year, she thought. In the beginning she'd started taking sleeping pills, as she had done previously, but as time wore on she found that the sleeping pills were working less and less and were often making her feel foggy the following day. She realised that taking sleep medication for such an extended period of time was probably not a great idea and she had resolved to get to the bottom of just why she found sleep so difficult to achieve.

Anne's family and friends had always thought of her as a worrier. Anne herself realised that she was always thinking ahead and trying to think of, and manage, things that could go wrong. Anne knew that sometimes her worries got her down a little but she didn't mind too much as she thought of them as a type of insurance. If she worried or thought about something sufficiently she believed she could plan for almost any contingency.

As her responsibilities at work increased and the juggle between family and work became more difficult there was even more that could go wrong and therefore more to worry about. Anne admitted that she was frequently feeling an overwhelming sense of dread that something truly awful was going to happen and she had to be ever-vigilant to prevent this unknown, but nevertheless catastrophic, event from occurring.

Anne had never thought of herself as having an anxiety issue. Sure, she was a worrier, and always had been but that didn't mean she was suffering from anxiety. She thought it even less possible that this was the cause for her sleeplessness. Once Anne understood that her worries (her anxiety) were indeed the cause for her sleep battles she began implementing strategies that allowed her to lessen her anxiety, which at the same time improved her sleep.

It is important to recognise that there is a wide spectrum of worry. Our worries may be minimal and reasonable. They may not even be directed at any one thing but just be a generalised feeling of worry that something is not quite right or that something may go wrong. On the other hand our worries can get out of control and become so great that they begin to affect how we go about our everyday activities and we begin to worry over minor things. For example, a boss's comment that there was a small error in the report you submitted becomes a vision of losing your job, a child's cold becomes concern that the child will die of pneumonia, and so on.

It often makes no difference whether our worries are reasonable or unreasonable – both will make relaxation difficult and cause sleep to become elusive. Once sleeping difficulties begin a vicious cycle can start to build up with our sleeplessness causing increasing anxiety which leads to increasing sleeplessness and then increased anxiety, and so on.

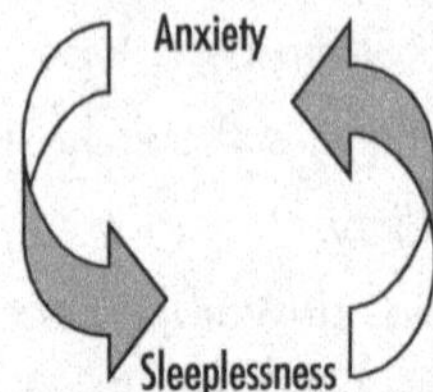

So how do you know if anxiety (or worry) is keeping you awake? While many of us may already know the answer to this question and are aware that, at some level, worries are keeping us awake, some people are unaware. The following questionnaire is a good way of quickly working out if anxiety is one of the causes for your insomnia so take the time to complete it now.

Over the last 2 weeks, how often have you been bothered by the following problems?	Not at all 0	Several days 1	Over half the days 2	Nearly every day 3	Score
1. Feeling nervous, anxious, or on edge					
2. Not being able to stop or control worrying					
3. Worrying too much about different things					
4. Trouble relaxing					
5. Being so restless that it's hard to sit still					
6. Becoming easily annoyed or irritable					
7. Feeling afraid as if something awful might happen					
TOTAL SCORE (add your column scores)					

Scoring: 0–4 minimal anxiety; 5–9 mild anxiety; 10–14 moderate anxiety; 15–21 severe anxiety.
Adapted from: Spitzer, R. L., K. Kroenke, et al. (2006). 'A brief measure for assessing generalized anxiety disorder: the GAD-7', *Archives of Internal Medicine*, 166(10): 1092–1097.

How anxious are you?

If you score 5 or above it may be that anxiety is causing problems with your sleep. Before we look at how to improve the situation it is firstly important to understand what it is about anxiety that causes us to have such bad sleep.

Something to think about

> If you score higher than 15 on the questionnaire it would be advisable for you to talk to your doctor as they will be able to offer you some specific advice that will assist you in addressing any problem you may have dealing with your anxious thoughts.

Anxiety activates our 'alert' hormones such as cortisol, adrenaline and noradrenaline. These are often referred to as the stress hormones because whenever we become stressed our body starts to increase their production, which in turn increases our blood pressure, heart rate and blood sugar levels. Ordinarily, this is a protective measure that allows us to be alert and to have more energy which better allows us to 'fight' the stress. Unfortunately though, our body will increase production of these hormones regardless of the source of the stress – whether it is in response to an imminent threat such as someone attacking you with a knife, or in response to a series of worrying thoughts.

The alert hormones also cause many other physical reactions such as muscle aches and tension, headaches, irritability, nausea, nervous energy, shortness of breath and sweating.

By understanding these physical reactions to our worries (or our anxiety) we can begin to understand just why worrying is so detrimental to sleep. In the previous chapter we looked at how the circadian rhythm of alertness works in harmony with the night hours and that during this time we experience a big drop in our alertness level, which allows us to fall asleep and stay asleep. If we are producing stress hormones late at night, however, they will cause us to become alert and prevent us from experiencing the drop in alertness so necessary for sleep. Simply put, the production of stress hormones actually prevents one of the essential processes of sleep from taking place.

What happens is that the alert hormones stimulate the alert pathways in our brain and prevent melatonin from working. The hormones that are produced in order to fight our stress wake us up and actively prevent us from succumbing to the sleepiness ordinarily induced by the melatonin. In this, these hormones are similar to the effects of caffeine. While caffeine effectively masks the sleep chemical adenosine and tricks the brain into thinking it does not need to sleep, the stress hormones mask the effects of the circadian rhythm of sleep and trick the body into thinking it needs to be alert.

In so doing, the body is only doing what it thinks is necessary. It would be extremely dangerous for us to feel sleepy or to fall asleep when we are in danger. Even though worrying thoughts mostly do not put us in danger they produce the same physical response and it is hard to get to sleep when our heart is racing, when we are breathing shallowly and when we have a lot of muscular tension. It is like getting out of the car with the motor running – the car might not be moving physically but the engine continues to run.

While we might feel a little concerned by the idea that worry is causing our sleeplessness, knowing that this may be the case is a good thing. Once we recognise that worrying can cause sleeplessness we can start immediately improving the situation because there are some good and simple techniques that we can implement that are highly effective at turning off our engine.

Chapter 6

Managing worry

IT IS ONE THING TO know that your worrying may be causing you to have sleepless nights but stopping those worries from intruding into the night-time hours can sometimes be difficult. It is, however, possible to train your brain to stay calm and look at life from a more positive perspective. Like training for physical fitness, training your brain to stay calm will take time and will require you to be vigilant in following particular practices. It would be foolhardy to expect that you could run ten kilometres after just a few days of fitness training and it would also be unreasonable to expect that good sleep will happen immediately.

In this chapter I will present four different techniques that will help you manage the stress hormones' response to anxiety and worry. You can use one, or a combination, of these techniques but make sure you choose one you are comfortable doing so that you will persevere with the training. So, read through each of these techniques, try them on for size and stick with the ones that work for you.

1. Understand exactly what you are worrying about

Many times we feel that our worries are caused by external events – for example, our partner, our children, or work issues. While the trigger may be external, the worrying process is internal and it is the dialogue within us that maintains the anxiety. When we're worrying, we usually talk to ourselves about things we're afraid of or negative events that might happen. Like Anne, we go over all the possible negative outcomes in our mind and think about all the ways we might deal with them. In essence, we try to solve problems that haven't yet happened or we imagine the worst-case scenario.

All this worrying may give us the impression that we're protecting ourselves by preparing for the worst. Anne thought this but then began to realise that all her worrying was only exhausting her and making her daily life difficult.

Sometimes worrying produces an effective solution and has been worthwhile. This is a 'productive' worry. But how do we know whether we have productive or unproductive worries? Perhaps one of the easiest ways to understand the difference is to do a direct comparison.

Helen's story

Helen and Jennie are both waiting for a train to get them to work. An announcement comes over the loudspeaker that the train has been delayed by at least an hour. Both Helen and Jennie have busy days planned and this delay will really affect their work schedules. Both immediately begin to worry and so their bodies start to produce the stress hormones adrenaline, noradrenaline and cortisol which increase their heart rates and their blood sugar levels (so they have more energy). They even may start to feel a bit hot and agitated.

Jennie realises very quickly that her boss will not be happy that she is late as they have a report due. Before Jennie calls her boss to notify her of the delay, she works out a way to ensure the report is completed on time: she can get her work colleague to get some information together so it is already waiting for her when she gets in and she can also organise an eat-in lunch. Jennie sets her plan in motion and all goes well. In this instance, Jennie's worries were productive and she was able to utilise all the stress hormones her body produced so that at the end of the day she felt tired, but relaxed.

Now compare this to Helen's reaction. Like Jennie, Helen knows her boss will not be happy if she is late as she too has a report due. Helen immediately starts to imagine that her lateness may make her boss really angry, so angry in fact that he might fire her. And even if he doesn't fire her for being late he will probably fire her because there is no way that she will be able to finish the report on time. Helen begins to feel nauseous and her head starts to ache. Unlike Jennie, Helen has been unable to use her stress hormones to implement actions and the more she worries about the situation the more stress hormones her body produces. By the time the train comes she is feeling highly agitated and fearful about how the day will turn out.

As it turns out though someone else from Helen's work was catching the same train and had notified a colleague about the delay. Helen's boss was not angry when she arrived and had, in fact, started work on the report. All Helen's worry had been in vain. It achieved nothing except to make her feel unwell for the rest of the day. By the time she got home that night she was still full of nervous energy and unable to get to sleep.

While this example clearly shows the difference between a productive and a non-productive worry, the distinction may not always be so obvious. If, however, you spend a lot of time focusing on 'what ifs' then it is highly likely that your worrying is unproductive. As a result, your body will produce a lot of stress hormones that increase your level of agitation and cause you to sleep badly that night.

By recognising unproductive worries we can start to deal with them in more productive ways. This may involve challenging irrational, worrisome thoughts; learning how to postpone worrying; and learning to

accept uncertainty in your life. We will look at some of the ways to do this in the next chapter.

2. Practise relaxation techniques

As we now know, our worries are more than just a simple thought because they result in a whole cascade of physical reactions. As we have learned, we begin to produce adrenaline, noradrenaline and cortisol in response to the perceived threat and so our heart starts to pound, we start to breathe faster and more shallowly, our muscles tense up, we get hot and we get a surge of energy. This is no problem if we can use these physical responses in a productive way, but what do we do if these thoughts are the 'what-if' type and are unproductive? Well, we can counteract the production of our stress hormones by actively relaxing.

Like worry, relaxation is more than a thought. It also produces a whole cascade of physical reactions. When we relax, our heart rate slows down, our breathing becomes slower and deeper, our muscles relax, and our blood pressure decreases. It is impossible to be anxious and relaxed at the same time and so improving our ability to relax is a powerful way of counteracting our stress responses.

There are a variety of proven ways that will increase your ability to relax but they require practice. Try to set aside at least 30 minutes a day to practise one of the techniques suggested below. This will increase your ability to relax and you will be less likely to experience a stress response to your thoughts. Over time, the relaxation response will become easier and easier, until it feels natural.

All of these relaxation exercises can be practised at any time during the day and especially at night, when we do not want any of our stress hormones keeping us alert and awake.

Progressive muscle relaxation

Before anxiety takes hold, progressive muscle relaxation can help release muscle tension and provide a time-out from worries. The technique involves systematically tensing and then releasing different muscle groups in our body. As our body relaxes, our mind will follow.

Progressive relaxation

This exercise can be done lying on your back on the floor. If lying on the floor is uncomfortable lie on your back on a bed.

1. Starting with the lower body and concentrating on your right side:
   (a) Squeeze your toes on your foot and point them downwards. Hold this position for 5 seconds then let go.
   (b) Flex your toes and pull them back towards your leg. Again hold for 5 seconds and then let go.
   (c) Straighten your knee, so that your leg is lying flat on the floor and tense your thigh and calf muscles. Hold for 5 seconds and then relax the leg.
   (d) Repeat each step on your left side.
2. Next move to your torso:
   (a) Squeeze your buttocks for 5 seconds and relax.
   (b) Tense your stomach and squeeze it in. Relax after 5 seconds.
   (c) Push your shoulder blades back and squeeze them together. Relax after 5 seconds.
3. Continue with the arms and face and hold each of the positions for 5 seconds. Make sure to relax before moving on to the next position.
4. Arms and shoulders:
   (a) Tense both hands to make fists.
   (b) Squeeze both arms into your sides.
   (c) Raise shoulders to your ears.
5. Face and neck:
   (a) Tense neck.
   (b) Purse lips.
   (c) Open mouth as wide as possible.
   (d) Wrinkle up nose.

(e) Squeeze eyes shut.

(f) Raise your eyebrows as high as possible.

Once you have completed this you should have a sense of lightness and definitely much less muscle tension. The effects of this exercise can be enhanced by visualising a relaxing location, like a beach.

Deep breathing

When we're anxious, we breathe faster and more shallowly. This causes symptoms such as dizziness, breathlessness and tingly hands and feet. These physical symptoms are frightening, leading to further anxiety. By breathing deeply from the diaphragm, we can reverse these symptoms and immediately calm ourselves down.

Deep breathing exercise

This exercise is easy to do and very relaxing. Try it any time during the day or night.

1. Sitting (or lying) in a comfortable position put one hand on your stomach just below your ribs and the other hand on your chest.
2. Take a deep breath in through your nose, and let your belly push your hand out. Your chest should not move.
3. Breathe out through pursed lips as if you were whistling. Feel the hand on your stomach go in, and use it to push all the air out.
4. Do this three to ten times. Take your time with each breath.

While continuing to keep one hand on your stomach and the other on your chest now:

5. Breathe in for a count of five.
6. Hold this breath for a count of seven.
7. Breathe out for a count of eight.
8. Repeat steps 5 to 7 until you feel calm.

Meditation

Many types of meditation have been shown to reduce anxiety. Mindfulness meditation is particularly effective and research shows that it actively reduces the production of the stress hormones.

Mindfulness meditation

This exercise is best done while sitting in a comfortable chair or on the floor. Make sure that your head, neck and back are straight but not stiff. If time is limited, set an alarm clock so that you can do this exercise without worrying about the time. If time is not limited set aside 20 to 30 minutes for this.

1. Try to put aside all thoughts of the past and the future and stay in the present.
2. Become aware of your breathing, focusing on the sensation of air moving in and out as you breathe. Feel your chest rise and fall, feel air enter your nostrils and leave your mouth. Pay attention to the way each breath is different.
3. Watch every thought come and go, whether it be a worry, fear, anxiety or hope. When thoughts come up in your mind, don't ignore or suppress them but simply note them, remain calm and use your breathing as an anchor.
4. If you find your thoughts getting carried away, observe where your mind went off to, without judging, and simply return to your breathing. Remember not to be hard on yourself if this happens.
5. As the time comes to a close (you will feel when you are ready to stop the meditation) or the alarm sounds, sit for a minute or two, becoming aware of where you are. Get up gradually.

3. Learn to recognise the stress response and counteract it

One of the things that is often most difficult for people to do is to recognise when they are experiencing the stress response. Often we are totally unaware that we are worried and our heart and breathing rate have increased, or that we have started tensing our muscles. Usually all we are aware of is a generalised feeling of agitation. If, however, we are able to recognise the telltale signs of the stress response we can start to actively counteract the physical reactions and begin to implement some relaxation techniques.

Believe it or not, research has shown that the key to switching out of an anxious state is to accept it fully. Almost counterintuitively, by accepting our anxiety we will cause it to disappear.

While this sounds relatively easy it often isn't. Frequently our worries plague us when we are trying to go to sleep or in the middle of the night. At times like these it may be useful to implement the strategy of AWARE. This stands for:

A: Accept the anxiety. It is important not to fight the anxiety but to accept it. If we resist it, we will prolong and increase the agitation that it brings. Our stress is not responsible for how we think, feel, and act and we can choose to think, feel and act differently.

W: Watch your anxiety. Look at it without judgement – recognise that your heart rate is increasing, that you are breathing more rapidly, that your shoulders are tense. Don't consider it good or bad, but rather just something that is happening with your body. Perhaps rate it on a 0 to 10 scale. By being detached you will be able to observe changes in these physical reactions. The more we can detach ourselves from the experience, the more we can just watch it.

A: Act with the anxiety. Pretend as if you aren't anxious, think some pleasant thoughts and make sure you breathe slowly and normally. By breathing normally you will be controlling the stress response and well on the way to decreasing its effects.

R: Repeat the steps. Continue to accept your anxiety, watch it, and act with it until it goes down to a comfortable level. And it will. Just keep repeating these three steps: accept, watch, and act with it.

E: Expect the best. What you fear the most rarely happens. A certain level of worry is normal and often beneficial in that it prompts us to do things we may be tempted to put off until tomorrow, but it's also important to think positively and expect good outcomes.

4. Adopt a healthy lifestyle

The importance of a healthy lifestyle in minimising anxiety and increasing the potential for good sleep cannot be overstated. What we eat and how we exercise affects how we think and how we sleep. A healthy, balanced lifestyle plays a big role in keeping anxiety under control.

It is critically important that we have healthy eating habits. We need to limit our caffeine and processed food intake and eat plenty of complex carbohydrates such as whole grains, fruits, and vegetables. Not only do these stabilise blood sugar, they also boost serotonin, a brain chemical with calming effects. Alcohol and nicotine need to be avoided at times of anxiety as both are stimulants and while they may seem calming they will lead to higher, not lower, levels of anxiety.

We also need to adopt a regular exercise routine. Exercise is a natural and effective anti-anxiety treatment. This does not mean you have to start working out strenuously for an hour every day. Far better that you undertake some regular aerobic activity for 30 minutes every day. This will not only relieve tension and stress, but it will also boost your physical and mental energy and sense of well-being due to the release of endorphins, the brain's feel-good chemicals.

As we will see in Chapter 16 healthy eating and exercise programs are not only important in managing our anxiety levels, they also play a role in the sleep process, so there is a very nice additive effect on sleep when we begin to adopt these healthy lifestyle practices.

Throughout this chapter we have concentrated on how to manage our stress response. Everyone encounters worry at certain times and it is to be expected. Learning how to manage it is therefore important for all of us whether we think of ourselves as a worrier or not.

The four techniques I have described in this chapter should be of assistance in helping us to sleep better whenever we are going through the more difficult times. At these times remember to:

1. Take the time to evaluate exactly what you are worried about and examine whether it is productive or not productive.
2. Practise one or more of the relaxation techniques suggested – progressive muscle relaxation, deep breathing or meditation.
3. Learn to recognise the stress response and to actively counteract it, perhaps by using the AWARE process.
4. Adopt a healthy lifestyle, exercising more and eating unprocessed, natural foods.

These techniques can be used individually or in conjunction with each other and will help to maintain a calmness that will minimise the stress response and allow you to achieve deep, restful sleep. However, it may be that while these techniques are useful they are not optimal for you personally. If this is the case you should spend some time researching various relaxation techniques as there will be one that will work well for you.

Chapter 7

Cognitive Behavioural Therapy

COGNITIVE BEHAVIOURAL THERAPY (CBT) IS highly effective at combating the feelings of anxiety that prevent us from relaxing and sleeping and can be used any time of the day or night. At the basis of CBT is the idea that a particular thought, or 'cognition', creates certain emotions that cause physical responses, which form how we behave. In other words, if we have a negative thought, we will have negative emotions and exhibit behaviour based on this negative emotion. CBT works simply by turning such negative thoughts, or negative cognitions, into positive ones.

We have already learned that each time we have an anxious thought we have a physiological response – we produce stress hormones, our heart rate and blood pressure increase and we may feel hot and agitated. While we may not realise it we also have a physiological response to a good thought – we decrease our levels of stress hormones, particularly cortisol, our heart rate and blood pressure go down and we feel relaxed and happy.

The idea behind CBT is therefore to teach us to think of alternative, more positive thoughts whenever we have an anxious, non-productive thought. In so doing we will cut short, or perhaps eventually prevent, the negative thought from happening and thereby minimise the amount of stress hormones in our body.

While the idea of changing a thought may seem a complicated process, it actually isn't and if we consider Maria's story we will understand much better how we go about changing our negative thoughts to positive ones.

Maria's story

On her arrival at work one morning Maria received an email informing her that her manager was coming to talk with her later in the day to discuss a project. Even though Maria had been working hard on this project there had been several set-backs and it was not as advanced as she would have liked. She immediately started to think that her manager would think her incompetent and that this would affect her chance of promotion. Maria started to worry and began to get quite agitated. By the time her manager arrived Maria was feeling sick and was on the verge of tears. She was almost unable to speak for fear of what was to happen to her and found it difficult to participate in the discussion.

What actually happened though was far from Maria's imagination. Her manager had come to compliment her on her continued diligence in working on a project that was facing so many barriers and to let her know that she was aware of set-backs and that she was happy with the progress that had been made. She wanted to discuss how to get the project back on track and was interested in Maria's ideas.

Despite the fact that, due to her stress, Maria found it difficult to think clearly in the meeting, she was relatively happy with the outcome and understandably relieved. By the time she got home she was feeling the best she had all day. Despite this happy outcome, however, Maria could not get to sleep that night and even when she did manage to get to sleep she did not stay asleep for long – waking up after only a few hours and unable to get back to sleep for a long time.

Maria constantly encountered days like these where she would feel sick and anxious about a particular meeting or project. Invariably though, everything turned out all right in the end and she would go home relieved that all was okay for now. Even though she would ultimately feel good about the outcome she constantly found sleep elusive and would often have considerable difficulty staying asleep.

Because we know already about the stress response we can easily understand why Maria felt sick and agitated by the thought of the meeting with her manager. By the time Maria went to bed her daytime concerns were long since resolved, yet she was still unable to sleep. The reason for this was that despite the resolution of her problem she had flooded her system with stress hormones during the day and unless she was able to actively dissipate them they would take some time to leave her system. Even if Maria's meeting with her boss had occurred in the morning it could still have affected her ability to sleep that night. This is why daytime stress can have such a devastating effect on our sleep.

Understanding this and learning how to combat it is where CBT comes in. In Maria's story she quickly jumped to the conclusion that her boss would find her incompetent. This immediately triggered a stress response, with adrenaline, noradrenaline and cortisol rushing through her body, increasing her heart rate and making her feel hot, sick and agitated.

If at this stage Maria had recognised what was happening to her she may have been able to implement one of the relaxation techniques or deep breathing exercises that we discussed in the previous chapter, which would have dampened her stress response. But instead she continued with her negative thoughts, so much so that by the time her manager arrived Maria was almost paralysed with fear.

Despite the happy outcome it was not surprising that Maria found sleeping that night difficult – there were still too many of the stress hormones in her system.

Maria needed to learn to recognise her stress reaction and try to actively counteract it with a relaxation exercise, but also to critically examine the thought (or cognition) itself and consider whether it was a reasonable thought. Maria needed to work out whether her thoughts were of the non-productive 'what-if' type, which were just increasing the level of stress hormones in her system, and if this was the case, to do something about it.

Maria could have reflected upon the fact that she had been employed by the company for the past 7 years, and had regularly received praise for her work and her work ethic. She could have also considered that the set-backs she had encountered with this project were outside her control, which had already been recognised by management.

If Maria had taken the time to make this reflection she may have well had an alternate, more positive thought along the lines of 'I have done a great job getting this project back on track after all the set-backs'. If Maria had been able to think like this she may have felt a little excited that the project problems were finally going to be tackled. Instead of all the stress hormones flooding her system, Maria would have experienced some of the feel-good hormones, which would have motivated her and allowed her to think clearly and positively.

The art of positive thinking

Sometimes when we are in the difficulty of the moment we may realise we are thinking negative thoughts but our minds have raced away so much it's difficult to start thinking a positive thought. In situations like this it is important that we at least recognise that we are having these negative thoughts, and if we cannot immediately replace them with a more positive thought, we should try a relaxation exercise, such as deep breathing or even practise a mantra (simply sounding the syllable 'Om' may quieten our thoughts sufficiently) so that we can begin doing CBT.

CBT is not a complex process but learning how to do it effectively can take some time and a considerable amount of self-awareness. Fundamentally it requires a number of steps. These steps and how they apply to Maria's situation are detailed in the following table.

If Maria had been able to change her negative thought to a more positive thought the outcomes would have been vastly different. Maria's story demonstrates how much our thoughts affect our emotions and

Step	Action	Maria's situation
1	Recognise the trigger (or situation)	The notification her manager was coming to see her
2	Recognise the automatic thoughts (or cognitions)	'I am incompetent' 'I am not going to get that promotion'
3	Recognise the emotional response to thoughts	Fear and nervousness
4	Evaluate physical response to emotions	Nausea, increased heart rate, agitation and inability to think clearly
5	Consider alternate, more positive thoughts	'I am a valued employee' 'This is an opportunity to work out how to get the project back on track'
6	Examine the emotional response to these new, more positive thoughts	Excitement, or happiness that problems may be resolved
7	Evaluate the physical response to these emotions	A renewed enthusiasm for the project Energy Clear thinking

how our emotions affect our physical reactions and behaviours. How right Shakespeare was when he wrote in *Hamlet* all those years ago: 'for there is nothing either good or bad, but thinking makes it so'.

Far better then, when possible, to think positively rather than negatively.

Keep in mind that the ability to do this improves with practice and it is never too soon, or too late, to start. The very next time you have an issue that causes you to worry take the opportunity to do some CBT – work out what the actual thought was that caused the initial concern and then critically analyse it to see whether there is another way of looking at that thought that is more positive and much less worrisome – then concentrate on going with that thought instead.

CBT can be practised anytime and anywhere. It can be used during the daytime hours to help us overcome negative thoughts as well as during the night hours. Successfully implementing some CBT techniques will certainly improve our stress levels and have a positive effect on our sleep, as we will see in the coming chapters.

Up to this point in the book we have spent considerable time examining whether anxiety is the cause of our insomnia and we have learned some techniques that will actively reduce anxiety. It may be tempting to think that all we have to do now is implement our newfound knowledge and all our troubles with sleep will be over. Unfortunately this is not the case. This is just the first step.

Next we will develop strategies to incorporate these techniques into a sleep plan for our particular type of insomnia. It is important not to rush in and think that we already know enough to get good, uninterrupted sleep. We need a little more information to apply to our individual situation.

Chapter 8

Getting to sleep

SLEEP-ONSET INSOMNIA, OR MORE SIMPLY, trouble getting to sleep at night, is a relatively common problem and often causes considerable stress. If you suffer from this you will be able to detect it very easily by examining your sleep diary responses in Chapter 4. Normally speaking, when a person does not have a sleep problem they will fall asleep within 20 minutes of lights out. Quicker than 10 minutes indicates that they are very tired, and more than 30 minutes indicates that either they are not tired enough to go to sleep or are unable, because of some other problem, to initiate sleep in a timely manner. People who suffer from sleep-onset insomnia can take up to 2 hours to get to sleep. For these people, instead of being a warm and inviting environment, bed is a battlefield where the nightly struggle to sleep takes place.

If you suffer from this type of insomnia you are not alone. Inability to initiate sleep is a common problem and it can have a number of different causes, including either a sleep disorder or anxiety. For the rest of this chapter we are going to concentrate on sleep-onset insomnia caused by anxiety. (We will discuss how to treat sleep-onset insomnia caused by a sleep disorder in a later chapter.)

For many people who have stressful lives or major worries, initiating sleep can present an enormous task, while for others it may just be the anxiety associated with going to bed (and the anticipated inability to get to sleep) that is the core of the problem.

In Chapter 7 we learned about Maria and the terrible day she had worrying about her manager thinking her incompetent. While the day had a happy ending, Maria could not get rid of her nervous energy and, despite feeling exhausted, that night she laid awake for a long time before falling into a fitful sleep. The next morning she felt so washed-out and unwell that she found going to work extremely challenging.

We know from the previous chapters that due to the excessive amount of stress hormones Maria produced during the day she had a heightened state of alertness and it was because of this that her body could not sleep. She had all the alert hormones in her brain and body and none of her sleepy hormones. It didn't matter how much she wanted sleep, Maria was not going to get it until she could lessen the amount of her alert hormones and increase her sleepy hormones.

Firstly, Maria needed to recognise that her stressful day was just that – a day that produced lots of stress hormones. Once she understood this she would have realised that she needed to implement some techniques to dissipate these hormones.

- She could have exercised a little – visiting the gym, or getting off the bus or train one stop earlier and walking an extra 20 minutes home. Once home she could have practised a relaxation technique, like deep breathing, while she prepared the evening meal. After dinner she could have sat down quietly, in a dimly lit room, and actively relaxed (using progressive relaxation) or undertaken a meditation exercise.
- If she still felt uptight she may have been advised to take a small amount of time (say 15 minutes) to write down what exactly was concerning her and possible solutions to these concerns.

If, despite undertaking these de-stressing activities, Maria could not get to sleep she could have got out of bed and moved to another room where she could have done some calming activity (like reading a magazine by lamplight) until she felt sleepy enough to try sleep again. If Maria had followed this strategy she would have been able to activate her off-switch, which would have enabled both her brain and body to get the rest they so desperately needed.

At this point you may well be thinking that this might be important information for Maria but what do you need to do to get over your particular problem of getting to sleep?

Well, as it turns out, the strategy suggested for Maria is what we should follow if we suffer from sleep-onset insomnia. The strategy can be summarised in the following steps:

Step 1: Assess your day

Many of us don't realise that what we do during the day can affect how we spend our night. There are numerous daily activities that can negatively impact our ability to sleep at night. Most of us are aware of many of these sleep-stealers: for example, we know that if we have a long sleep in the afternoon we will have trouble getting to sleep that night; or if we have too much coffee we will find sleep difficult. What many of us with sleep difficulties fail to realise, however, is that if your day has been stressful (like Maria's day), unless you do something to dissipate all the stressful hormones that have built up in your body during the day you will have problems getting to sleep and often problems staying asleep.

Step 2: De-stress

If you have had a stressful day like Maria then it is important you actively find ways to decrease the amount of stress hormones in your body. This could be as simple as taking the dog for a walk or doing some gardening. Time and again studies have shown the essential role exercise plays in sleeping well – the more exercise the better the sleep. By exercising we not only exert our bodies physically but we also reduce our stress hormones and produce some wonderful feel-good hormones. Care does need to be taken, however, not to exercise within 3 hours of bedtime, and ideally before 6 pm as strenuous exercise can alert the body.

If, after doing some physical exercise, you still have not managed to decrease your feelings of worry, follow Maria's example and take 15 minutes to write down what you think might be causing you to maintain this level of anxiety. Once you have written this down use some of the techniques described in the previous chapters to deal with the issues. For example, you might want to do a step-by-step CBT exercise and think of alternative, more positive thoughts, or you may examine these thoughts to see whether they are productive or non-productive, and deal with them accordingly.

Step 3: Work with your sleep process (and not against it)

Essential to overcoming any type of sleeplessness is an understanding of the sleep process itself. If we remember back to chapters 3 and 4 there is almost an ideal period when we can get to sleep within a reasonable amount of time. Critical to this is our understanding of our own, individual cycles. In Chapter 3 you were asked to track your feelings of alertness throughout the day, which should have given you your pattern of alertness. If you haven't done this yet, you should do it now as it is important in helping you develop your customised sleep schedule.

Most people will find that their peak of alertness is before 11 pm and will find the processes set out below very useful in helping to get to sleep within a reasonable time. If, however, after completing your alertness cycle you discover that you are one of those people who have a late peak of alertness (after 11 pm) then you may in fact be suffering not just from worrying thoughts but also from something called Delayed Sleep Phase Syndrome (DSPS). This syndrome is a recognised sleep disorder and needs special attention. We will discuss this in a later chapter, but you will need to follow the steps we are discussing now as well.

The vicious circle

Sometimes when we suffer from sleeplessness we try to catch up on our sleep by going to bed early, often before our evening peak of alertness. This is counter-productive. Going to bed too early will mean that we will end up staying awake for longer and not be able to get to sleep until our alertness cycle is in the downward direction. This inability to get to sleep when we want to often causes a stress response, which only prolongs our inability to get to sleep.

Knowing when our peak of alertness occurs allows us to know when it is time to start preparing for sleep. For example, if your evening peak of alertness is around 9 pm, it is at that time that you can start doing the things that will enhance your ability to go to sleep. These include:

1. Making sure that you are exposed to dim lighting as this will kick-start the production of melatonin essential to consolidated sleep.
2. Putting away all electronic equipment and resisting the temptation to stay on the computer. This applies also to mobile phones and tablet devices – anything that emits a bright light.
3. Ceasing any work or study so that your brain starts to reduce the activity of the wakeful pathways.
4. Doing one of the relaxation exercises described in Chapter 6 – meditation, progressive relaxation, or deep breathing. If you enjoy yoga then do that; be aware though that any practice, be it yoga or meditation, must be relaxing and not physically active, otherwise it may keep you awake. These relaxing practices will also reduce muscle tension, a signal to the brain that it is time to sleep.
5. Taking a warm to hot shower. If we recall that we fall asleep more readily on a decreasing body temperature, we can easily see why this might promote our sleep pathways. A warm to hot shower increases our skin temperature and when we cool down after the shower we enhance our already naturally decreasing temperature, thereby reinforcing the message that it is time to sleep.

By following these five processes we reinforce our natural 24-hour cycle of alertness (or sleepiness) which will make it much easier for our brain to go to sleep naturally.

Step 4: Follow good sleep practices

Good sleep practices are often referred to collectively as good sleep hygiene. While there are many practices recommended for good sleep there is a core group that should be adhered to at all times to ensure deep, restful sleep.

Adhering to these practices is fundamental to good sleep for everybody and they are discussed in a chapter of their own – Chapter 15.

It is imperative that you read this chapter and understand why these practices are essential to getting good sleep.

Step 5: Go to bed only when sleepy

In Step 3 we discussed how we needed to work with our cycle of alertness and only try to sleep after we had passed our evening peak of alertness. This step is an extension of that.

Feeling sleepy is different to feeling tired. While we may frequently use these words interchangeably, sleepiness has its own set of behavioural characteristics such as yawning, drooping eyelids, nodding off to sleep while watching TV, and so on. By recognising these telltale signs and using them to our advantage – by going to bed when we experience them – we should fall asleep fairly quickly.

While this works well for some people, for others, waiting until they feel sleepy has limited impact because as soon as they go to bed and attempt sleep, their mind (and body) wake up immediately. People often describe this like a light bulb being switched on – all of a sudden, despite the fact they had been finding it hard to stay awake while watching TV or reading a book, sleep becomes extremely elusive and they feel awake and alert as soon as they try to go to sleep. For these people sleep is frequently associated with negative thoughts. Because in the past they have found getting to sleep so difficult the mere act of going to bed can evoke the stress response which immediately makes sleep elusive. If this is you then you need to pay attention to the next step.

Step 6: Get out of bed if you don't fall asleep within 30 minutes

As we now know, it is normal to take about 20 minutes to fall asleep. Much longer than this indicates that either we are not tired enough to fall asleep or we are having trouble initiating sleep. In either case we need to get out of bed. This may not be easy because if we are tired we like the idea of being in bed. We are also often optimistic and think that we will be able to get to sleep soon, and by getting out of bed we are denying ourselves this opportunity. This is far from reality. When we lie in bed, awake, we often start to think all those negative thoughts such as 'I am never going to get to sleep', 'Why is sleep so hard?', and 'I won't be able to survive tomorrow unless I get to sleep now'.

The more of these thoughts we have the greater the stress response and the more elusive sleep becomes.

To break this cycle we need to get out of bed and wait until we feel sleepy again. When we do get up we need to ensure not to undertake any activity that will wake us up even more, such as switching on the computer, having a cup of coffee, or smoking a cigarette. Instead we need to make sure that we are in a dimly lit room, perhaps reading a magazine under lamplight. This is also an ideal time to practise some CBT and think alternate more positive thoughts about sleep or about what went on during the day, or practise some deep breathing or relaxation. Once we start to feel sleepy again (yawning, eyes drooping) we can go back to bed and try to get to sleep. If again we become alert and cannot fall asleep within a reasonable time period then we need to repeat the exercise until we naturally fall off to sleep. It may be for the first night or two we will need to do this a number of times, but this will definitely lessen over time.

A word of advice: make sure you do not clock-watch as this too will frequently promote a stress response – 'Oh no, it's already midnight and I am not asleep yet!' Instead, approximate the time period and use your innate knowledge of yourself to recognise when you no longer feel sleepy or inclined to sleep. It is at that point that you need to get out of bed.

For many of us this will sound rather tedious and it may take quite some time for things to improve, but be resolute. Things will start to improve over a period of a few days because what we are doing is gradually decreasing our anxiety around sleep and hence the stress response – the more we do this the more the processes of sleep will dominate over the alert pathways (which have been promoted by the stress response) and the quicker sleep will come to us.

Step 7: Get out of bed at the same time every day

One of the problems faced by people who have difficulty sleeping is that when the alarm finally does go off in the morning they are reluctant to get out of bed and will take the opportunity to sleep in. For anyone suffering sleeplessness this only serves to exacerbate an already difficult situation.

People who struggle with sleep have what can be considered 'fragile sleep' – everything and anything can cause a disturbance to their sleep.

Consequently, establishing a routine is of primary importance. By setting a fixed getting-up time we are training our body to stop our sleep processes at that time and to start with the alerting processes. If, when we get out of bed, we expose ourselves to bright lights or even 5 minutes of deep breathing or stretching, we will enhance the awake pathways and actively assist in the process.

When the body gets used to a routine of waking up at say, 7 am every day, it can start putting in order all the other biological activities including, most importantly, the daily rhythm of alertness (and sleep). When this happens it creates the harmony of processes that we discussed in Chapter 3. For fragile sleepers, a sleep-in means a delay in the body clock and ultimately an inability to get to sleep that night.

The importance of keeping to a set time of waking in the morning cannot be over-emphasised. Even in people with no real sleep problem, a disruption in the sleep processes is commonly seen as a consequence of a Sunday morning sleep-in. All too often, people who sleep in on Sunday will find it difficult getting to sleep Sunday night and wake up Monday morning tired and unrefreshed – a phenomena now often referred to as 'social jet lag'.

So even though you may feel tired when that alarm goes off, make sure you get up and, if you can, expose yourself to some bright light (sunshine if possible) and some light exercise. You will certainly reap the benefits of doing this when you find yourself able to get to sleep more easily that night.

By following the steps set out in this chapter, our ability to initiate sleep should improve over time. If we feel success is not coming quickly enough we need to keep in mind that we have experienced difficulty falling asleep for a considerable period and have undoubtedly built up a whole series of bad sleep habits that can only gradually be changed. While we may wish it to be different, it does take time to change habits that have taken half a lifetime to develop.

Chapter 9

Staying asleep

TROUBLE STAYING ASLEEP, OR SLEEP-MAINTENANCE insomnia, is a common problem and frequently occurs in combination with experiencing difficulty getting to sleep (sleep-onset insomnia). This is because some of the same disruptions of sleep processes are involved but can affect people in different ways. I have separated sleep-onset problems from sleep-maintenance problems, and treated them as if they are entirely different, but in reality this is often not the case. If you suffer from both types of sleeplessness it is important that you pay heed to the solutions for each of the problems – this will give you the best chance of overcoming your sleep problems.

Sleep-maintenance insomnia is diagnosed when a person finds that they wake up after only a few hours of sleep and are unable to get back to sleep for hours; or when a person wakes up many times throughout the night never feeling like they get to deep and refreshing sleep.

If you have either of these problems then you have sleep-maintenance insomnia. You will readily be able to confirm this by looking at your sleep diary. If you have noted multiple awakenings or one long period of wakefulness a few nights a week and you wake up feeling very tired then you have sleep-maintenance insomnia. It doesn't matter whether it takes one form or the other, the end result is the same: instead of getting the 7 or 9 hours of sleep you crave, you end up with only 5 or 6 hours – leaving you tired and unrefreshed, and at risk of all the ill-consequences we spoke about at the beginning of the book. The good news is that we can develop a pattern of good solid sleep with minimal wakeful periods.

Before we go into how to improve sleep-maintenance insomnia we firstly need to understand the issues a little bit more. According to research, sleep-maintenance problems are frequently suffered either when a person has anxiety or when they have an undiagnosed sleep disorder. As both of these problems have their own specific set of therapies we will deal with them separately. For the rest of this chapter we will discuss the particular effects of anxiety on the ability to maintain sleep and will look at sleep disorders in later chapters. It is of course possible to have both anxiety problems as well as a sleep disorder and be unaware that both these issues are denying you good sleep, so while reading this chapter keep in mind that if you have been told you snore or move a lot in bed, you need to pay special attention when you get to those chapters dealing with these disorders.

Causes of sleep-maintenance insomnia

To begin to understand the problem of sleep maintenance it is necessary to have some knowledge of the processes that normally allow most of us to sleep for a consolidated period of 7–9 hours every night. We looked at these processes in chapters 2 and 3 and learned that the ability to sleep for an uninterrupted period of time was the synchronisation of our sleep drive (our need for sleep) with a number of our 24-hour biological rhythms (circadian rhythms) such as our temperature cycle, our melatonin secretion and, most importantly, our alertness cycle. We also learned in those chapters that we cycle through different stages of sleep and that these cycles included brief periods of wakefulness.

It may come as a surprise but our modern-day pattern of sleeping for a consolidated 7–9 hour period is a relatively new phenomenon. Up until about 250 years ago, prior to the Industrial Revolution, the majority of people were rural workers and they spent a lot of time in dark hours. Once the sun went down access to light was limited and expensive so people were exposed to dim light for a longer period than we are today.

It appears that in this pre-industrial world there was a two-stage (or biphasic) pattern of sleeping, whereby people went to sleep 1–2 hours after sunset and slept for several hours (referred to as the first sleep) before getting up around midnight. They would then spend the next hour or so awake, read a little (by candlelight), make love, talk with neighbours, before going back to sleep until sunrise. This did not mean that these people suffered from insufficient sleep. Far from it. They still managed to get an average of 8–9 hours of sleep, it was just that it was in two sleep periods. Indeed even today, research has shown that when humans are exposed to increased dark periods (up to 16 hours) they will adopt this biphasic pattern. This pattern of sleeping makes sense because, if we recall that once our eyes are exposed to fading light we start to produce our sleepy hormone of melatonin, it is not surprising that we would naturally fall asleep a few hours after the light started to fade. When we manage to get away from all the bright city lights, for example, when we go camping, most of us notice that we get tired much earlier and tend to go to sleep earlier than when we are at home. In these circumstances many of us will wake with the dawn. This is a natural way of sleeping and is in keeping with our cycle of melatonin production.

Notwithstanding its more natural pattern, the biphasic sleeping period seems to have disappeared around the time of the Industrial Revolution when there was a big migration from the farm to the city and when working in the daylight hours was extended to working in the night hours. Presumably this was because the 10-hour period required for this biphasic pattern of sleeping was no longer available in the busy world of factories and trade. This meant that the 1 hour or more of wakefulness in the middle of the night had to be done away with, allowing people to consolidate the two sleeping periods into one long sleep.

While this consolidated pattern of sleep works well for many of us today, it would seem for others that the wakeful period during the middle of the night may indeed be an evolutionary throwback that reflects a more natural pattern of sleeping.

This means that if you do experience a wakeful period in the middle of the night, it may not be the consequence of some other problem, but rather a natural phenomenon. The problem arises of course, when you *want* to sleep and can't. In our modern world we are expected to sleep in one consolidated time block. When we don't do this most of us will become anxious about getting the sleep we need and the very fact of this anxiety, with its consequent stress response, means that we stay awake for a long time. So what starts as a natural phenomenon ends up causing a big problem.

In these circumstances we have to learn to accept the wakeful period, recognise it as a natural phenomenon and not be concerned about it. In this way we will be able to fall back to sleep quite naturally, without becoming hot and bothered in the meantime.

If you think this more natural type of sleep may be the cause of your night-time wakefulness then practising some CBT will definitely help. Instead of the negative thought of 'Oh no I am awake again and I won't be able to get back to sleep' leading to the negative stress response, we can think 'This is a natural pattern of sleeping and I will naturally fall back to sleep. I might as well use this time to think about pleasant things in my life.' Fortunately happy thoughts will stimulate the feel-good hormones (in the same way as negative thoughts stimulate the stress hormones) and enhance our ability to fall back into sleep.

Sometimes though, a prolonged period of wakefulness in the middle of the night is not the consequence of a natural sleep pattern. When we cycle through sleep during the night we experience multiple brief periods of wakefulness. These brief periods of wakefulness should be just that: brief. Indeed, the majority of us do not remember them at all. For others, what is meant to be a quick transit through wakefulness wakes them up and they cannot get back to sleep for a considerable time.

This sustained wakeful period may be the result of a stressful day (like we saw with Maria) or may be a consequence of a 'learned' stress response to waking up during the night. While the underlying process is the same – alert hormones causing sleep to disappear – how they come about is different.

If we recall Maria's story in Chapter 7 we will remember that her stressful day caused her a sleepless night. This was due firstly to her inability to dissipate the high levels of stress hormones her body had produced during the day. As a result, even though she managed to eventually get to sleep (due to her high sleep drive) once her sleep drive decreased a little she was vulnerable to being woken up – which happened when she transited through what should have been a normal brief period of wakefulness. At this time in her sleep cycle, because she still had high levels of stress hormones, she was alerted into full wakefulness. Once this happened and Maria realised she was fully awake, the secondary anxiety process began – she became more stressed because she realised she was awake and started to worry about her ability to get back to sleep – which of course produced even more of the stress hormones, and hence sustained wakefulness. When this happened Maria had to wait until her sleep drive increased sufficiently to allow her to get back to sleep.

Maria's story is by no means unusual and all of us have had nights like hers when just the simple act of waking up can cause us to stay awake for hours worrying about not sleeping. If this happens often enough, it can become a learned response and whenever we experience a brief, wakeful (and normal) period during the night we are at risk of becoming fully awake due to the learned stress response, even when we have no other stress in our lives. This is often the cause of chronic sleep-maintenance insomnia.

The other type of sleep-maintenance problem – when we experience multiple awakenings throughout the night – is often a result of some ongoing anxiety that we may or may not recognise, as we can see when we read Michael's story.

Michael's story

Michael is a radio program producer. He works very long days and spends a lot of his time in high stress situations trying to keep the program to time and dealing with difficult and unpredictable problems. Since his marriage broke up about 2 years ago he has been going through a complex property settlement and it does not look like this will resolve any time soon.

Michael has been having problems with his sleep for most of his life but it has become particularly bad over the last year or two. He realises his lack of sleep is affecting both his professional and personal life and he is finding it increasingly difficult to keep up with the hectic pace of work, especially as his organisational skills seem to have disappeared. He has recently found that he is working longer hours because he can't seem to get through his work as efficiently as before and he regularly doesn't get home until 7.30 to 8 pm. When he does get home he nearly always feels stressed so he normally has a glass or two of wine to help him relax. He admits that he may be drinking more than is good for him. On the personal front he is constantly having arguments with his children and ex-wife and often finds himself being abrupt and annoyed with his friends.

Michael usually manages only between 5–6 hours of sleep each night despite trying hard to get more. Generally, because he is so tired, he goes to bed around 10 pm and falls asleep quickly. More often than not though, despite his extreme tiredness, he wakes about 1.5 hours later and then for the rest of the night he is in and out of sleep, waking every hour or two and staying awake for a variable period each time. By the time he wakes up at around 6 am he is exhausted by the effort of trying to stay asleep.

As we know brief periods of wakefulness are normal and are seen even in those who get consolidated sleep. Michael's periods of wakefulness though (shaded in grey on the diagram on the next page), are not brief (they can last up to an hour) and they are numerous. Occasionally he manages a good night of sleep, but this is unusual and he is not sure why this is the case. Michael feels like he has tried every sleep tip in existence but none of them have helped.

Michael does not consider that the cause of his sleeplessness is worry. He does recognise that his personal life has caused some stress but he is dealing with it well and it certainly doesn't keep him awake at night (or so he thinks).

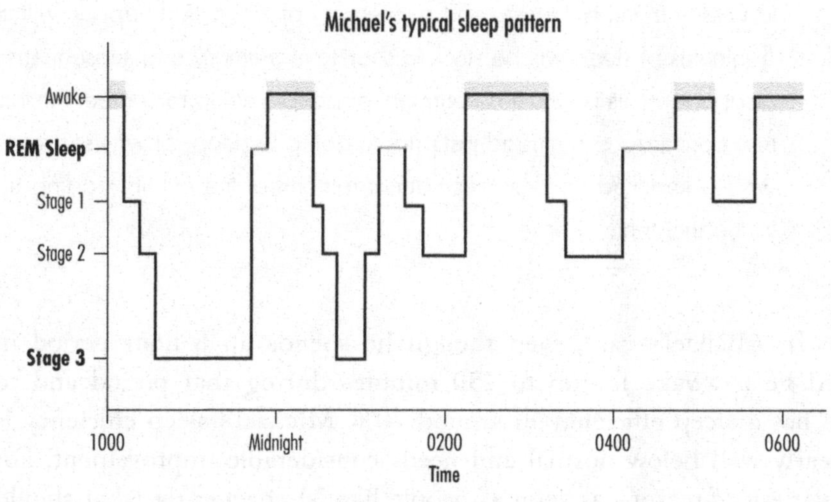

By unravelling Michael's story we can begin to work out ways we can overcome the problem of night-time awakenings.

When we have problems staying asleep one of the things that is often evaluated is something called sleep efficiency. This is the measure of the time spent in bed, wanting to be asleep, compared to the total amount of sleep we actually manage to get. Ideally, for the well-slept person, we aim for a sleep efficiency of about 95%. This means that even very good sleepers should expect to spend at least 5% of their total sleep time awake. For example, if we sleep for 8 hours (480 minutes) it is normal to spend up to about 20–30 minutes awake. This wakefulness is mostly not remembered because if it is for less than 5 minutes at a time it is too brief to be consolidated into our memory. So even though the well-slept person has these brief awakenings they do not recall them the next morning.

Did you know?

For something to be remembered it must be stored in long-term memory. When we first learn something it is held in short-term memory, and when we actively reinforce it, it will be transferred to long-term memory. When we sleep, the door between the short-term and long-term memory closes, and so memory of things that happen within 5 minutes of sleep will be stuck in short-term memory and subsequently disappear. This is why it is common for people not to remember the last few paragraphs they read just prior to going to sleep, or why someone who is knocked unconscious cannot remember the events leading up to the incident.

In Michael's case, even though he spends an 8-hour period in bed he is awake for up to 150 minutes during that period and so he has a sleep efficiency of around 70%. Michael's sleep efficiency is clearly well below normal and needs considerable improvement. For a variety of reasons as soon as people like Michael enter what should be a brief period of wakefulness when they transit, for example from REM sleep to NREM sleep, they become fully alert and remain awake for an extended period of time. It may be that they are particularly sensitive to noise or light and as soon as their partner starts to snore or some light enters the bedroom they wake up and become alert. Unfortunately for these people, because this has happened so often they begin to worry about whether they will get back to sleep, which immediately stimulates the stress response and makes sleep elusive.

Michael's problem was not a sensitivity to light or noise but rather, in common with many other people who lead stressful lives, he had not taken the time to adequately deal with his worries during his awake time and consequently had to deal with them in the night hours when he wanted to be sleeping.

Most of us have busy lives and there will be times when we have to contend with extra pressures. Even though Michael considered that he was coping with everything well he did not realise the effect his marriage break-up and divorce settlement was having on his daily life (and sleep).

Michael luckily did not suffer from sleep-onset insomnia. He had such a big sleep debt that as soon as he went to bed he fell asleep, but no matter how tired he was he generally woke 1–2 hours after going to sleep and then was in and out of sleep for the rest of the night.

By examining Michael's day we can see how the stress was impacting on his sleeping. Normally Michael got home from work around

7.30–8 pm. As he was often in bed by 10 pm this gave him little time to manage his stress. After he had a few drinks and his dinner, he spent some time on the computer dealing with his personal affairs and then he would shower and go to bed. Nowhere in his routine was there any down time! Like so many of us, Michael was going to bed wanting to sleep for the next 8 hours without ever bothering to switch off his mind or his body. In other words, he was getting out of the car but forgetting to turn the motor off. As a result, even though he fell asleep quickly the moment he entered into what should have been a brief wakeful period his 'motor' jumped into action and he sprang to wakefulness. Once awake Michael would begin to worry about his ability to get to sleep again, further exacerbating his inability to sleep.

How then to break this awful cycle and get Michael to have the sleep he wants and needs? There are a number of strategies that Michael was able to implement that considerably improved his sleep and which enabled him to get consolidated sleep most of the time. The strategies he adopted make up the steps you can follow if you have difficulty staying asleep. Some of these steps are the same as the ones we can follow if we are having trouble getting to sleep at night, but they are equally as important for allowing us to stay asleep for a consolidated period so I will mention them again here, even if only briefly.

Step 1: Assess your day

As we saw in the previous chapter it is important to reflect upon our day and to recognise when it has been stressful and to realise that we need to actively work on decreasing our levels of stress hormones. The importance of this first step cannot be over-emphasised because it is consistently one of the things we fail to do. Perhaps the easiest and best way to de-stress is to do some exercise, like a 20-minute walk with a friend or taking the stairs instead of the elevator.

If, despite doing some exercise, you still do not feel sufficiently calm take 15–30 minutes to write down what you think might be causing you to maintain this level of anxiety. We have already discussed this idea in the previous chapter, so perhaps, if this is an issue you deal with, it would be worthwhile to revisit that section. Don't forget also about the importance of relaxing the mind and body and preparing it for sleep by doing any of the things we have already discussed like a relaxation exercise, deep breathing or meditation.

Another way to stop our stress hormones is by having fun. This solution is frequently overlooked as many of us spend so much time being stressed that we fail to realise that if we started having fun we would feel so much better. When we experience fun our brain stops producing the stress hormones and starts to produce all the feel-good hormones. So enjoying ourselves, laughing and generally having a good time predisposes us to good sleep. This is why so often people who sleep very poorly during the working week report sleeping well on Saturday night, a night traditionally associated with fun and relaxation.

So try and factor some fun thing into your day or night. This does not have to be complicated and can be as simple as phoning a friend, watching a funny movie, or reading a book you enjoy. Whatever it is, provided you find it enjoyable, you are promoting your feel-good pathways which are so essential for deep, restful sleep.

Step 2: Follow good sleep practices

Good sleep practices are absolutely essential to good sleep and are discussed at length in Chapter 15. It is important that you pay close attention to, and stick to, these practices so please make sure that you read that chapter with care. In the meantime though, if you suffer from sleep-maintenance insomnia there are two things that are particularly relevant to your sleep practice.

Firstly, caffeine is a big culprit for the inability to stay asleep. All too often people who have poor sleep use caffeine to counter-balance both their anxiety and tiredness. While it might seem that caffeine is helping it truly is not. Caffeine has a long half-life and can stay in our system for up to 7 hours. This is especially so if you are over 45 because as we age our metabolism slows and it takes our body longer to process the caffeine. This means that, even though we may have a cup of coffee at 9 pm, for some of us caffeine will still be in our body as late as 4 am.

Many people who have trouble staying asleep do not recognise that their caffeine consumption may be an issue. This is because they have no trouble falling asleep – indeed many can fall asleep almost immediately and so they think that their after-dinner coffee is not to blame. If this is you, then take heed. If we are still under the effects of caffeine when we go to bed we may, because we are so very tired, be able to get to sleep fairly quickly. Once our need for sleep reduces a little (which it will do while we are actually sleeping) and we go through a normal period of transiting through wakefulness, the presence of caffeine in our system will immediately stimulate us into wakefulness and we will have trouble getting back to sleep until either the caffeine is sufficiently metabolised or our need for sleep is so strong that we will fall back into sleep.

The problem of caffeine also plays out against the background of other problems. For example, as soon as we can't get back to sleep we start to worry about not getting to sleep which results in the stimulation of stress hormone production, or as soon as we are awake the stresses of the day that we have not adequately dealt with now come front of mind and we end up evoking a stress response. So be aware: if you drink coffee or have any caffeinated drinks or food, make sure that you restrict these only to the morning hours.

Secondly, alcohol could be causing our sleeping problems. If you are experiencing any difficulty sleeping then alcohol is definitely not recommended. People are often surprised by this as they associate drinking alcohol with sleepiness. Indeed, while alcohol has an initial sedating effect, it is rapidly metabolised and after 4–5 hours there is minimal blood alcohol remaining. After this time the person experiences what is known as 'rebound wakefulness' which can mean periods of shallow sleep and multiple awakenings, sweating, increased heart rate and overall general activation (as opposed to the normal quietness associated with sleep). So rather than increasing sleep, alcohol actually reduces total sleep time.

Step 3: Sleep restriction

People suffering from an inability to stay asleep commonly spend a lot of time during the night trying to get to sleep, which is indicated by their sleep efficiency. As we saw with Michael, his sleep efficiency was around the 70% mark when what is needed is around 95%. If we have trouble staying asleep then an effective way to increase our sleep efficiency is to practice sleep restriction.

Sleep restriction aims to improve our sleep efficiency by limiting the amount of time we give ourselves to sleep in bed. It is based on the idea that the less time we sleep the greater our sleep drive and our need for sleep. For example, if we stayed up all night tonight (maximising our sleep drive, or need for sleep) and tomorrow we only gave ourselves 3 hours of sleeping time, chances are that we would probably sleep for the entire 3 hours – giving a sleep efficiency of 100%. Sleep restriction therapy works in the same way but on a less extreme level. As we increase our sleep drive our sleep becomes more consolidated and our sleep efficiency improves.

Successfully practising sleep restriction involves a stepwise approach and needs to be continued until we are managing to sleep the desired number of hours and sleep efficiency is around 90–95%.

1. In Chapter 4 there is a sleep diary that hopefully you have filled in over a week-long period. If not, this first step has to wait until you have recorded 7 days of sleep. Once you have kept the diary for 7 days, add up the number of hours you slept each night. This is the number recorded in the column 'Last night I slept for a total of . . .' Once you have the total number of hours divide this by 7 to work out your nightly average. For example, for Michael, the total number of hours he slept was 38 hours in the week, divided by 7 days gives us 5 hours 24 minutes. This is Michael's average sleep time. You will probably have noticed that you sleep more on some nights than on others, so it is important to get the overall average for one whole week and not just for one night.
2. We now need to work out our sleep efficiency. To do this, add up all the hours that you spent in bed each night during the week. This is the number recorded in the sleep diary column 'Last night I was in bed for a total of . . .' For example, Michael regularly went to bed at 10 pm and got out of bed at about 6 am every morning, which means that he was in bed for a total of 8 hours each day, so 56 (8 x 7) hours a week.

   Once we have worked out the total hours spent in bed, we need to calculate sleep efficiency by dividing the number of hours slept per week by the total number of hours spent in bed. To bring this to a percentage we simply multiply by 100. This can be more simply written as:

$$\text{Sleep efficiency} = \frac{\text{total hours spent asleep in one week}}{\text{total hours spent in bed in one week}} \times 100$$

Doing this calculation for Michael:

$$\text{Sleep efficiency} = \frac{38 \times 100}{56}$$
$$= 68\%$$

Knowing our average sleep efficiency is important because this is the measure that we want to see improve each week.

3. We now work out our going-to-bed and getting-up time. If we need to be awake and up by 7 am to get to work and our average sleep time as calculated in step 1 above is 6 hours then we *do not go to bed* until 1 am. This means that we are only giving ourselves a total of 6 hours in bed each night (which is our calculated nightly average of sleep time). By doing this we should improve our sleep efficiency.

   It is important that the wake-up time is maintained and that when our alarm goes off we do not linger in bed trying to get more sleep. This new schedule now needs to be maintained for one week and it is vital that we keep a sleep diary for the entire week. Without this record we will quickly forget how well (or poorly) we are sleeping and it will be difficult to detect small improvements. For Michael, as he sleeps on average 5 hours and 24 minutes and needs to be up at 6 am every day his going-to-bed time for his first week was calculated at 12.30 am.

   In the first few weeks we often experience difficulty keeping awake until the scheduled bedtime, so we need to be prepared and have some interesting books to read or DVDs to watch. We may also feel much more tired during the day than usual and, if this is the case, we need to take advantage of a quick nap – keep in mind, no more than 20 minutes – during our afternoon lull (if you don't know when this is go back to Chapter 3 and complete your cycle of alertness).

4. At the end of the first week we go through the same steps and work out both our average sleep time and sleep efficiency

and compare these to the ones calculated the week before. For Michael his average sleep time for the week was a little less, 5 hours 10 minutes, but his sleep efficiency had greatly improved to 93%. This meant that, even though for that week he had slightly less sleep, he was actually sleeping for most of the time he was in bed.

If after restricting our sleep time for one week there is an improvement in our sleep efficiency so that it is greater than 80% then the time we spend in bed can be increased by 30 minutes. For Michael this now meant that he was able to go to bed at midnight while still maintaining his 6 am awake time. If by the end of the week we have not managed to increase our sleep efficiency to above 80% we are still allowed to increase our time in bed by 30 minutes if we spend less than 45 minutes awake during the night.

For the next week we must maintain this new bedtime, again making sure that we get up as soon as the alarm sounds. At the end of this second week if there has been a sustained improvement in sleep efficiency, or an improvement in the amount of time we spend awake during the night, we can again increase our total sleep time by 30 minutes. In the case of Michael he was able to go to bed at 11.30 pm in the third week, and because he maintained his sleep efficiency of 93% this meant that for the first time in 12 months he was getting more than 6 hours consolidated sleep.

5. We need to keep repeating the above steps each week for as long as it takes to get to our ideal sleep time, while at the same time having minimal awakenings. Don't increase sleep time if sleep efficiency does not improve (or goes backwards). Don't worry, it will improve, but it does take more time for some than others.

   If we become a bit stuck and our sleep stops improving before we reach our ideal sleep pattern it might be an idea to implement the next step.

Step 4: Get out of bed if you are still awake after 30 minutes, even if it is 4 am

One of the issues with nightly awakenings is that they can last a long time and can cause all sorts of anxious feelings to bubble to the surface. We need to get up if we do not get to sleep within 30 minutes; so too do we need to get up if we are awake for 30 minutes or more in the middle of the night. This is not an easy thing to do because we normally try to be optimistic and think that we will soon be able to get to sleep, and if we get out of bed we will never get to sleep. As we have already discussed in the previous chapter, however, this is not the reality because the longer we lie in bed awake, generally the more anxious we become. Far better to break the cycle, get out of bed and only go back to bed when we feel sleepy again. As cautioned previously, when we do get up we have to be careful not to do anything that will increase our alertness, so we need to make sure that we are in a dimly lit room maybe reading a book or doing one of the relaxation exercises already described. When we start to feel sleepy again we should go back to bed as going to sleep this time will be much easier.

If, however, we continue to feel anxious about our ability to sleep and sleep is proving very elusive it is time to read the next step.

Step 5: Practise CBT

For many of us suffering from sleep-maintenance insomnia, CBT is an effective tool. It is the rare person who, after having many nights of interrupted sleep, does not wake up once again without that feeling of dread and thinking 'here we go again'. If this sounds familiar then practising CBT can prove to be helpful.

For more about how CBT works you can read Chapter 7 and Chapter 14.

Step 6: Maintain the same getting-up time

When we are practising sleep restriction this step is vital, but it must be maintained even when we get to the stage of sleeping through the night without wakening. It needs to be a lifelong habit because establishing a routine is of primary importance. Even though we may feel tired when that alarm goes off, we must make sure that we get up and, if we can, expose ourselves to some bright light (sunshine if possible) and some light exercise.

By following the six steps set out above our problems with sleep maintenance should improve over time. As would be expected the turn-around will not be immediate, but with practice and diligence, sleep will improve. Indeed within about 5 weeks Michael was managing to get the sleep he wanted most nights and was coping much better with his work and his personal issues.

Being disciplined about something that should come naturally may seem odd at first, but it is necessary. We are retraining our body to be in harmony with all its processes and, unless we are diligent, this will not happen. So do persevere – things will improve with the disciplined approach.

The good news about Michael

Despite the fact that Michael was initially very sceptical about the idea that his problems with sleep were caused by the combination of his stressful work life and personal issues – a sort of overwhelming of his system with stress hormones – he was prepared to give the steps a go because he was desperate to get better sleep.

He began firstly by getting off the train one stop earlier and walking the rest of the way home. While he was walking he started thinking about some of the issues he had confronted during the day and thought about some potential solutions. Once he got home he physically let go of his work environment by changing out of his work clothes. He then spent about 15 minutes writing down some of the thoughts that he had on his walk home and importantly he wrote down in his 'worry book' what he thought might be solutions for the issues. He then put the book away.

His nightly routine also changed. He no longer opened a bottle of wine when he started preparing dinner – in fact he decided only to have a glass of wine when he was around friends. After his dinner he made sure to factor in something fun – normally he watched a funny movie or read a novel – something he hadn't done in years. He also made a decision to spend only 30 minutes on his computer, because if he didn't do this he ended up spending much more time in front of the screen and didn't have enough time to factor some enjoyment into his evening.

He followed the sleep restriction process and found that, especially in the first weeks of sleep restriction, he had much more time in the evenings (in his first week he was not allowed to go to bed before 12.30 am) and so a few times in that week, and the following weeks, he made plans to go out with some friends. This again was new for him as before he was always so tired he would refuse social engagements as he just wanted to go to sleep.

He also made sure to prepare his mind and body for sleep. One hour before his set bedtime he would make sure he was in a dimly lit room, practising a relaxation routine – his favourite was a 15-minute meditation. This was something he had done in his younger days but had been forgotten about when he had children.

Before he went to sleep he made sure to think about how CBT could help him if he woke during the night. As a result he became much less likely to worry if he did wake up and, at such times, if he was awake long enough he would use that time to either think about some enjoyable plan or, just in case he thought he would be very tired the next day, he would work out a way that he could get in a 20-minute sleep in his lull period the next afternoon – which seemed to significantly calm his worry about not getting enough sleep.

Although he did not need to, Michael also agreed that if he was awake for more than 30 minutes he would get out of bed, and do some quiet activity in a dimly lit room until he was feeling sleepy again. Once he started implementing all the new practices his sleep began to improve markedly. Within 5 weeks Michael was getting the sleep he wanted and coping much better with his work and his family and friends. Michael felt for the first time in a while that life was pretty good.

Chapter 10

Waking up too early

WHEN PEOPLE WAKE UP EARLY in the morning, at around 4 am, and no matter how tired they are they just cannot manage to get back to sleep, this is called early-morning-awakening insomnia.

This can be the result of a number of different processes including the problem of only *thinking* that we wake up early, because unknowingly we mistake being awake with being asleep. While this at first glance may seem impossible it is more common than we realise and especially so in the early hours of the morning when we are in and out of our light sleep. When this happens it is referred to as sleep state misperception and it happens in both good and bad sleepers, although it occurs more frequently in people who have insomnia. As sleep state misperception is more correctly classified as a primary insomnia we will speak more about it in Chapter 14.

Sleep state misperception is not the only cause of early-morning-awakening insomnia. Frequently this type of insomnia is associated with an advanced circadian rhythm and often, when we examine the history of people who have this, we will find that they have always gone to bed a little earlier than everyone else and have been habitual early risers. Although in the past this may not have caused any real issue, problems may start to emerge as we get older. As we age, if we keep both physically and mentally active, our need for sleep remains fairly constant from about age 30 onwards – we still require between 7–9 hours each night. What does change, however, is the structure of our sleep and it is common for our circadian rhythm of alertness to advance in our older age. As it advances many of us will begin to go to bed earlier and to wake earlier. While this is mostly unproblematic for those of us who in younger days had the circadian rhythm of an owl (going to bed late and getting up late) it can become very troublesome for those who are natural larks. For these people, who have always greeted the day a little early, they start to greet the day earlier and earlier, so that eventually they will be in their awake zone around 3.30–4 am and they find it almost impossible to return to sleep.

This would not be so much of an issue if bedtime was at 7.30 pm. However, because most of us like to stay up and spend time with family and friends, bedtime is often not until 9.30–10 pm. If this bedtime is maintained, along with the early morning awakening, it means that it is only possible to get 6–6.5 hours of sleep each night and in this situation sleep deprivation will quickly ensue along with all the concomitant ill consequences.

Josh's story

For as long as Josh could remember he had loved getting up early. Even as a teenager he had found it difficult to be asleep much after 6.30–7 am. In this he was much like his father and, because the two of them were often awake before the rest of the household, they would go surfing or fishing and get back home just as his mother and sisters were getting out of bed.

When Josh grew up he continued to be an early riser, which suited him as he was a builder and normally needed to leave home around 5.30 am to start work about 6 am. For most of his working life Josh had gone to bed around 9 pm and got up around 4.45 am. Josh was now 52 and for the last year or so he had been having a lot of trouble sleeping much past 3 am. This meant that with his 9 pm bedtime he was only averaging around 6 hours every night and he was feeling exhausted. Although sometimes he managed to get to sleep earlier, it was difficult because the family normally didn't eat dinner until about 7.30 pm and then he liked to spend some time with his wife and children.

Josh's constant wake-ups at 3 am were really getting him down. He realised that he was becoming difficult to live with because he felt more stressed about everything and he found himself being easily irritated with his co-workers and family. On top of all of this he had now lost interest in sex.

As a way to become more relaxed in the evening, Josh had started drinking more than he had in the past. He had always enjoyed a glass of wine with his meal, but he rarely had more than one. Now he was finding that he sometimes had three or even four glasses of wine because he felt more relaxed afterwards. While he thought that this may not be the best solution to his problems, he was at a loss to know what else to do.

He had spoken to his doctor about this problem and she had mentioned that sometimes drinking and early morning awakenings can be a sign of mild depression. Since he had none of the other signs she did not think this was the case though. Josh was pretty sure he was not depressed either but he really needed help getting his sleep back on track.

Josh was certainly in a bad way and quite desperate for a solution. He was hoping for a magic bullet to fix his sleeping problems. Luckily for him his doctor recognised that while sleeping pills might solve his immediate need for sleep in the short term, they were not a long-term solution and that Josh needed to work at getting his sleep pattern back in order.

From Josh's story we can see a few common issues that cause sleeping problems. Firstly, as Josh had grown older his natural lark tendencies had become exaggerated and, instead of the natural rhythm of his day being 5 am to 9 pm, his internal body clock had advanced so that his natural rhythm was probably more likely to be 3.30 am to 7.30 pm.

As Josh found it almost impossible to go to bed at 7.30 pm it meant that his internal body clock was in conflict with his external social clock.

Sadly, Josh had exacerbated the situation by increasing his alcohol intake. As we have discussed before, while alcohol initially has a sedative effect it is actually a stimulant that is rapidly metabolised by the body. After 4–5 hours there is minimal blood alcohol remaining in our body at which time we will experience what is known as rebound wakefulness. For most of us, who do not have Josh's early morning body clock, this means that after this 4–5 hours we will experience periods of shallow sleep and multiple awakenings for the rest of our sleep period.

For Josh this meant that from about 2 am onwards, due to his alcohol intake, he was in a lighter sleep than normal. Unluckily for Josh his body's alarm clock was already set to wake him at 3.30 am, and because he was in light sleep at this time he was easily aroused. As a result he ended up being fully awake unable to fall back to sleep for the rest of the night, night after night. What complicated this situation even more is that Josh had also developed an anxiety about his early morning awakening, and so whenever he woke up he had a negative thought, 'Oh no, I am awake again and won't be able to get back to sleep', which further worsened what was already a bad situation.

The good news is that Josh's sleep can be improved, but as with the other types of chronic sleeplessness it will take time and require discipline.

Something to keep in mind

Although early-morning-awakening insomnia is often associated with an early-timed circadian rhythm it may also be due to depression. Often it is difficult to tease out whether the depression is a result of the lack of sleep or whether the inability to sleep is consequent to the depression. If you are not naturally a morning person, or if you have just started waking at 4 am unable to get back to sleep, it may be that you have depression and need to consult with your doctor about this. While it is important that you do speak with your doctor it is equally as important that you continue to work on improving your sleep pattern.

Step 1: Stop drinking alcohol

The first thing Josh had to do was stop drinking in the evening. He found this more difficult to do than he expected because he had begun to rely on the alcohol to help him feel better. Rather than stop altogether he decided to gradually reduce his alcohol intake and each week he drank one less glass a night than he did the week before. This meant by week 4 he was not drinking at all.

Step 2: Exercise and get exposure to bright light in the early evening

Once he started to reduce his alcohol intake, the next thing that Josh needed to do was try to delay his body clock. Ideally he needed to shift it back so instead of waking at 3 am he could again start to awake around 5 am. In order to achieve this shift Josh had to alter his evening routine.

Firstly, he needed to incorporate some exercise in the early evening, preferably outside in the light. This is definitely not recommended for those of us who have the more usual body clock timing, but it was exactly what Josh needed. By exercising at around 7pm he will wake his body up and start producing more of the alert hormone cortisol, which promotes the alert pathways and actively prevents us from falling asleep.

The exercise had the added bonus of helping Josh complete step 1 because the exercise decreased Josh's stress hormones and increased his feel-good hormones, which meant he didn't feel like drinking. After his evening exercise, Josh then had to ensure that he was kept exposed to bright lights – strong kitchen fluorescent lights are good for this. This is important because exposure to bright lights delay the secretion of melatonin – our sleepy hormone and the hormone that sets our body clock schedule. By doing this we are able to push our body clock back. While bright fluorescent lights work well enough there are now portable bright light therapy devices available on the internet that are proving to be effective. These have bright lights embedded into an optical frame and watching TV or reading a book is still possible while wearing the device. The device needs to be worn for about 50 minutes prior to going to bed so Josh tended to wear the device from about 8 pm onwards.

For Josh, the combined effect of bright light therapy and evening exercise worked well and after 3–4 days he was waking up about

15 minutes later. Over the next few weeks as he continued with the bright light therapy and no alcohol regime he continued to shift his body clock back so that by the end of Week 4 he was again waking at 5 am.

Step 3: Practise CBT

While Josh was slowly resetting his body clock he was still waking up much earlier than he wanted. Although he tried not to, he was still having negative thoughts about his sleep so that when he woke early his first thought would be 'Oh no, here I go again, I am not going to be able to get back to sleep', which he now knew would kickstart his stress response.

Josh was keen to stop this negative thought process, and to optimise his chances of getting back to sleep when he woke too early, so using his knowledge of sleep he started to develop alternate more positive thoughts about his sleep such as:

'My sleep is better today than it was yesterday and it will be even better tomorrow. I know now how to improve it.'

'My early morning awakenings are just part of my natural cycle and it is not because I am doing anything wrong.'

'If I am really tired today I can have a quick 20-minute nap mid-afternoon.'

'Waking up at this time is part of the sleep cycle and it is normal to have brief awakenings.'

As Josh began to feel better about his sleep he was able to notice other things about his physical response to waking early. He became aware that when he woke at this time sometimes his muscles would start to tense. When this happened he knew he was decreasing his chances of falling back to sleep so, along with some CBT, he started doing the active relaxation exercise. Even if he didn't manage to fall back to sleep he felt much better for doing it.

Step 4: Minimise exposure to early morning light

People like Josh, who suffer from an advanced setting of the internal body clock, will always be inclined to wake early. If they are not careful they can unknowingly advance their body clock. They do this by exposing themselves to early morning light.

Every body, when exposed to morning sunlight, stops producing melatonin and is alerted into full wakefulness. As soon as this happens the body clock starts to tick down so that by the time 15–16 hours pass the body will be ready to sleep again. If, after a few days, we do not stop the early morning light exposure, we will have effectively advanced our body clock – and find ourselves waking up that little bit earlier naturally. While this may prove advantageous for the owls amongst us (who sometimes wake up later than they would like) it is certainly something the larks need to guard against – otherwise they will end up like Josh, waking at 3.30 am.

Once Josh had started setting his body clock back he had to be on the alert for this happening to him, so he made sure that he was not exposed to bright light in the morning hours for as long as possible and he started wearing dark glasses on his way to work.

Step 5: Do not nap in the afternoon

Finally, Josh had to guard against having a long afternoon sleep. For anyone encountering any type of sleeplessness the 2-hour afternoon sleep is extremely counterproductive as it just allows us to continue with our bad habits. Josh was therefore encouraged whenever he felt like sleeping for a few hours in the afternoon to follow this specific procedure which allowed him to have a little, well-timed nap, but did not interfere with his night-time sleep:

1. Because caffeine is a stimulant but takes about 30 minutes to work into our system, Josh had a cup of coffee about 3 pm.
2. He then lay down for an afternoon nap, and just to make sure, he set an alarm to wake him 20 minutes later.
3. Invariably he would fall asleep very quickly (apart from his tiredness due to his early morning awakening, it was also the time of his afternoon dip in alertness).
4. By the time his alarm went off 20 minutes later the stimulating effect of the caffeine was beginning to work so Josh was able to get up feeling much less sleepy and more alert than when he had gone to sleep. Importantly, this amount of sleep did not interfere with his sleeping at night.

By following these steps Josh's sleep improved and after a few weeks he was able, most mornings, to sleep until about 5 am. He now realised that he had an in-built early morning alarm clock and he would need to be vigilant about his sleep habits and not disturb the timing of his body clock in any way. The good thing was that if he ever inadvertently disrupted his body clock he was confident that he would be able to turn things around and get his sleep back into order without too much trouble.

The one other thing that may have helped Josh get his sleeping pattern back on track was melatonin. Short-acting, compounded melatonin can be effective in helping re-align the body clock. In Australia this is available by prescription and should be taken under the guidance of a doctor as timing the dosage is critical to its efficacy. If melatonin is taken at the wrong time it can actually advance the body clock even further, rather than helping to delay the time of awakening.

Having discussed many of the aspects of why we may not be able to initiate or maintain sleep, it is now time to turn our attention to some other causes of secondary insomnia and see what can be done about these in order for us to achieve good, consolidated sleep.

Chapter 11

Sleep disorders

MANY OF US (ABOUT 40% IN FACT) **complaining of problems with sleeplessness have at least one sleep disorder that has not been diagnosed. This is a real shame as most sleep disorders are easily treated and can lead to an improvement in sleep quality fairly quickly. Unfortunately people can go for years without being diagnosed, often resulting in significant professional and personal consequences.**

Paula's story

Paula was a high-performing banking executive. She was 52 years old and felt like she had not had a good night's sleep for years. She was constantly exhausted and overwhelmed by the simplest of tasks. For the last 10 weeks she had been off work, having decided to take her long-service leave to try to improve her health. She had expected her sleep problems to improve when the stress of work had abated, but hadn't experienced any relief.

When asked, she thought that perhaps her tiredness had started about 10 years ago. At that time she was finding it hard to stay asleep and would often wake up in the early hours of the morning and stay awake until it was time to get up. She had been prescribed an antidepressant, and while that gave some relief, over time her fatigue, depression and general lack of motivation had only increased. Her personal life was also suffering and her long-term relationship had ended, due partly, she thought, to her ongoing depression and lack of motivation. On top of this her general health was steadily deteriorating and she had just been diagnosed with type 2 diabetes.

When I met her she was at desperation point. It did not take long to work out that Paula's problems were the result of an undiagnosed sleep disorder – sleep apnoea. Once this was diagnosed it was easily treated and within a very short period of time (a week) Paula was feeling almost like her old self and ready to take on the challenge of returning to work.

Sleep disorders range from the very mild to very serious. There are so many recognised sleep disorders (eighty-five are listed in The International Classification of Sleep Disorders) that it is beyond the scope of this book to detail them all. In this and the next chapter I will focus on those that are considered most problematic and feature most often in the problem of sleeplessness: restless legs, circadian rhythm disorders and sleep apnoea.

Sleep disorders are commonly not recognised – either by the patient or their doctor – or misdiagnosed due to the difficulty of understanding the symptoms. The symptoms of a sleep disorder can be broadly divided into two groups: those that occur during the day (including excessive tiredness, headaches, mood swings, lack of energy); and those that occur during the sleep hours (including snoring, pauses in breathing, twitchy legs, sleep-walking). While we are aware of the daytime symptoms (we are tired or grumpy), we generally are unaware of our night-time symptoms as we are asleep. Even if we wake up briefly as a result of the sleep disorder, for example we wake ourselves up snoring, it is unlikely we will remember the event as we don't consolidate it in our long-term memory.

This means that what we report to our doctor is our daytime symptoms (sleeplessness, poor mood state, morning headaches) and not our night-time symptoms. As a result the doctor may treat the presenting symptoms (tiredness, depression) with a sleeping pill or antidepressant prescription, but may fail to diagnose the *cause* of the symptoms. This means that the cause of the presenting symptoms, say restless legs or sleep apnoea, can go untreated for years, all the while continuing to cause disrupted sleep and often condemning the person to a lifetime reliance on medication. Constantly treating the symptom is a lot like treating a leaky radiator by topping it up with more water. Doing this will definitely solve the problem in the short term but if we never fix the leak it will only deteriorate over time.

So, if you think your sleeplessness may be the result of an undiagnosed sleep disorder pay close attention to this and the next chapter. If, after reading about the disorder, you think it describes your problem then you need to consult with your doctor as soon as possible – because there are real solutions. On the other hand, if you think you may have a sleep disorder but don't think it is any of the ones described in these chapters, I recommend that you speak with your doctor as soon as possible so that a diagnosis can be made and treatment undertaken.

Movement disorders

Restless Legs Syndrome (RLS) and Periodic Limb Movement Disorder (PLMD) are sleep disorders characterised by movement during sleep. While both are movement disorders there are some major differences: in RLS the movements occur both during the day and night, are voluntary and in response to uncomfortable sensations; in PLMD movements are involuntary and only occur when a person is asleep. Both RLS and PLMD have a major impact on sleep and many patients report difficulty falling asleep or staying asleep due to the unpleasant limb sensations. This in turn causes extreme daytime fatigue, which is often the presenting symptom. People may or may not be aware of the movements during sleep.

Restless Legs Syndrome

RLS is one of the most common sleep disorders and is thought to affect about 22% of those people who struggle with sleep, although it remains largely undiagnosed. RLS primarily affects the legs, but may be felt in the arms as well. People experiencing RLS describe it as unpleasant 'creepy, crawly' sensations that occur in the legs when they are sitting or lying still. Symptoms are generally alleviated by movement – stretching, getting up and walking around or massage – and it is this constant need to stretch or move the legs that prevents the person with RLS from achieving and maintaining sleep.

Therese's story

Therese lived in a small country town. While she enjoyed living there she also loved the fact that she had always been able to escape to her beach house some 3 hours' drive away and so it was a big disappointment that she could no longer drive herself there. Over the past 5 years Therese had started suffering from dreadful insomnia and she was always exhausted. She had also developed a type of neuralgia which made sitting for any long period of time intolerable. She described her neuralgia symptoms as 'insects crawling on my skin' and for years they had caused her much discomfort. She would frequently delay going to bed because she knew the sensations would increase when she was lying down. She often woke at 3 am needing to walk around the room to get some relief. She frequently did not go back to sleep after this time and if she did she only ever slept fitfully. Apart from the neuralgia she had also been diagnosed with anxiety and early-morning-awakening insomnia as a consequence of her discomfort. She had been prescribed antidepressants as well as sleeping pills.

Despite these medications, Therese continued to have dreadful sleep and her life became restricted. It was with considerable relief that Therese found out that she had RLS and that it was treatable. Within a short time she was able to travel to the beach house again and resume all her previous activities. Moreover, her anxious disposition improved and she no longer required antidepressants or sleeping pills.

Unlike many other sleep disorders, the symptoms of RLS do occur in the awake hours, although they are most noticeable during periods of inactivity – long car trips, sitting, reading or studying. Consequently they are more commonly perceived in the evening when activity slows down. RLS symptoms also worsen in the evening and during sleep, presumably because in addition to inactivity there is a generalised decrease of motor activity associated with the sleep process which makes the sensations more noticeable.

RLS can profoundly affect daily living. Apart from the extreme fatigue brought about by lack of sleep – which has all the cognitive, behavioural and metabolic consequences that we have spoken about – people with RLS are often reluctant to undertake anything that involves a period of inactivity such as long trips, attending long meetings, going to concerts, and so their lives can become quite restricted.

Before a diagnosis of RLS is made four essential criteria need to be established.

1. The patient has an urge to move the legs (and sometimes the arms), usually accompanied by, or caused by, uncomfortable or unpleasant sensations in the legs.
2. The urge to move or the unpleasant sensations worsen during periods of inactivity.
3. The urge to move or the unpleasant sensations are relieved or partially relieved by movement such as walking or stretching.
4. The symptoms are worse in the evening or night than during the day, or they only occur in the evening or night.

Once diagnosed, RLS is easily treated. As it is often associated with a variety of other medical conditions, treatment depends upon the underlying cause. More and more evidence is emerging, however, that in many cases there is a brain iron deficiency causing the RLS. In these circumstances something as simple as oral iron supplements will improve symptoms, as was the case with Therese. Once RLS was diagnosed, Therese's doctor measured her iron levels and ferritin stores and found them to be on the lower end of normal. She prescribed Therese supplemental iron and within about 6 weeks Therese's symptoms began to lessen and within 3 months she had stopped taking her anti-depressants and sleeping pills.

RLS is about twice as common in women as in men and, while it used to be thought of as a condition of middle age, it is now becoming apparent that RLS may actually start at a younger age, but remain undiagnosed until middle age. Retrospective studies indicate that many adults diagnosed with RLS recalled symptoms beginning during adolescence – when it is usually labelled as 'growing pains'. Given this, it is an interesting fact that more than half of children diagnosed with Attention Deficit Hyperactivity Disorder (ADHD) have been shown to have RLS and that treatment with supplemental iron improves the behaviour in many of these children.

Periodic Limb Movement Disorder

The other type of sleep movement disorder that can unknowingly cause insomnia is Periodic Limb Movement Disorder (PLMD). PLMD usually occurs in the legs but can also affect the arms. The movements do not occur continuously throughout the night but are episodic and tend to cluster in the first half of the night when NREM is greatest. PLMD usually consists of a rhythmic extension of the toes, together with an upward bending of the ankle, knee or hip.

As periodic limb movements tend to cluster in the first third of the night, the person with PLMD will often struggle to get to and/or maintain sleep in this earlier part of the sleep period. In these cases they may well be diagnosed with sleep-onset or sleep-maintenance insomnia and be given a sleeping pill to assist in sleep onset, which treats the symptom rather than the cause. Alternatively, even if the person is not fully awakened by the movement they will still suffer severe daytime fatigue as they will be unable to get consolidated sleep. This is because the movements cause repetitive momentary awakenings (of which the person is unaware) resulting in a lot of light sleep (stages 1 and 2 NREM) and not the deep restorative sleep we all need. In both cases, the person suffering from PLMD invariably experiences substantial fatigue that can severely affect their daytime functioning.

PLMD is diagnosed during an overnight sleep study but there may be a simpler way to know whether we may have this or not. While we may not be aware of our movements, our sleeping partner invariably is. So if our partner tells us that we are a very restless sleeper and move a lot, or if morning after morning our bed looks like a battlefield, then it may be that we have a sleep movement disorder such as RLS or PLMD. As both of these disorders can be easily treated it is important that we talk about this with our doctor.

If we do find out that we suffer from either PLMD or RLS and have it treated many of us will almost immediately notice an improvement in our ability to get to sleep and to maintain our sleep. For some of us, however, the turn-around will not be so immediate. Due to the fact that we have suffered sleep problems for many years, some of us will have developed either an anxious disposition towards our sleep or have built up a raft of sleep practices that are counter-productive now that the underlying sleep problem is being effectively treated.

This means that once we are treating the sleep disorder we will need to turn our attention to Chapter 15 and make sure we are following all the advice given there. We may also need to go back over the chapters on stress and anxiety and make sure that we are not unknowingly allowing the stress response to continue to interfere with our sleep. If this is the case practising some CBT and developing alternate more positive thoughts in conjunction with RLS/PLMD therapy will enable us to get our longed-for sleep.

Circadian rhythm disorders

In Chapter 3 we talked about our circadian rhythms and how important they are in achieving good, consolidated sleep. In that chapter we learned about larks and owls and how our in-built circadian alertness cycle affects our time to bed and our getting-up time.

In Chapter 3 you were asked to complete your own cycle of alertness profile that would help you determine whether you were a lark or an owl. Hopefully you did this because, apart from the insights it gives you about your daily cycle of alertness, it is also essential information for determining whether or not you are an extreme lark or an extreme owl – both of which can have enormous consequences for your ability to sleep at either the beginning or at the end of the night.

Charlotte's story

Charlotte was only 17 years old and already she was having terrible problems with her sleep. When she was younger she used to sleep very well but over the last year or so her sleeping pattern had incrementally declined. She was now in her final year of high school and facing tough exams. She knew that she was not performing at her peak; she was always tired and was often totally unmotivated to do any study whatsoever. All she wanted to do was sit around and do nothing.

Charlotte really wanted to get good marks and she knew that if she was to do this she needed to get more sleep. The very fact of her not sleeping was making her more and more anxious and depressed about the pending examinations. Unfortunately for Charlotte, even though she was truly very tired during most of the day, she seemed to come alive at night and never felt like going to sleep until at least 1 am. As Charlotte had to get up every morning around 7 am to get to school this meant that she was only averaging about 5–6 hours' sleep per night. Many mornings she would get to school and just sleep for the first few lessons, to the considerable annoyance of her teachers.

On weekends, Charlotte would spend a lot of Saturday and Sunday sleeping. She would get up around midday and feel the best she had all week. On the weekends she didn't bother to go to bed until about 1.30–2 am and on these nights she fell asleep easily. Her parents couldn't understand what was going on and thought she was being a difficult (and lazy) teenager.

Charlotte had seen her doctor and had been told that her anxiety regarding her academic performance was preventing her getting to sleep and she had been prescribed antidepressants to help with this anxiety. This had helped a little but Charlotte continued to battle to get to sleep before midnight and so she, her parents and her teachers were desperate for some resolution to her sleep problem.

If we recall all that we have learned about the importance of circadian rhythms it doesn't take much investigation to work out that Charlotte is probably an extreme owl and that her internal rhythm of alertness is not allowing her to get to sleep at a 'normal' hour. As her late sleeping hour bumps up against the imperative of a set wake-up time it means that she is chronically sleep deprived and suffering all consequent cognitive and mood effects.

Charlotte's extreme owl nature was confirmed when she did her alertness profile over a few days. She found that at 11 pm and midnight, she was feeling wide awake and not at all inclined to go to sleep. Her alertness cycle was not just out in the evening but also in the morning when she recorded between a 3 (fighting sleep, wanting to lie down) and a 5 (somewhat foggy, let down) on the alertness scale until 10–11 am. This was the reason why she just wanted to sleep during her morning classes. It was no wonder that Charlotte was really struggling.

In sleep medicine terms Charlotte suffers from Delayed Sleep Phase Syndrome (DSPS). People with this experience a phase delay of their sleep–wake cycle of between 2–5 hours. This means that instead of being able to go to sleep between 10 pm and midnight (which would normally allow for 7–9 hours of sleep depending on wake-up time) people with DSPS cannot fall asleep until between 1–4 am, which normally results in severe daytime fatigue, unless of course they can consistently sleep in the next day. Luckily though, once asleep, people with DSPS have normal sleep quality and if they go to bed at their delayed hour they have no trouble falling asleep. In adolescents DSPS is often associated with daytime irritability and impaired school performance, and in adults very poor job performance and relationship difficulties. Those who have this disorder suffer chronic sleep deprivation with all its consequent problems including poor mood state, lack of motivation and so on and not surprisingly, left untreated, these people may be mistakenly diagnosed with depression.

DSPS is fairly common (and largely undiagnosed) in the younger age group and affects about 7% of adolescents and young adults (up to around 30 years of age). It is much less common in middle age (about 1%). DSPS is more prevalent in the younger age group for two main reasons. Firstly, around puberty the circadian cycle is lengthened and instead of averaging 24 hours it is more likely to average 24.3 hours, with some adolescents experiencing a circadian cycle of up to 25 hours. Secondly, it would seem that around puberty there is a greater sensitivity to any shift in melatonin secretion so that if there is any delay in melatonin secretion (say, due to a bright light source or high level of activity) then it is much more likely to reset the body clock.

Undiagnosed, the combination of the longer intrinsic day with the increased sensitivity to melatonin can cause an enormous amount of suffering for the young person, and for the 1% of adults who continue to experience this throughout their lives.

As we age our circadian cycle advances, which is why most sufferers of DSPS tend to improve as they age.

This is also why most people prefer to go to bed a little earlier as they grow older and are more inclined to wake earlier. As we saw in Chapter 10 where Josh started waking up early every morning, this can become a problem if the phase advance is too great and we become an extreme lark. This is the complete opposite of Charlotte's problem as these people's body clocks are advanced by 2–5 hours so they may wake as early as 2 am. In sleep medicine terms these people have Advanced Sleep Phase Syndrome (ASPS).

ASPS is rare in young people, affects about 1% of middle-aged adults and increases with age. Due to the early waking it is often diagnosed as depression especially where social demands, as in Josh's situation, do not allow for the earlier bedtime.

Both ASPS and DSPS are a recognised cause of sleeplessness although often, because the presenting problem with DSPS is sleep onset (and therefore likely to be confused with anxiety) and with ASPS it is early morning awakening (and therefore likely to be confused with depression), they are largely undiagnosed in general medical practice and frequently need specialist diagnosis.

Once diagnosed both disorders are relatively easily treated. The aim of the therapy is to try to bring both the advanced and the delayed phases to the typical sleep phase as illustrated in the diagram.

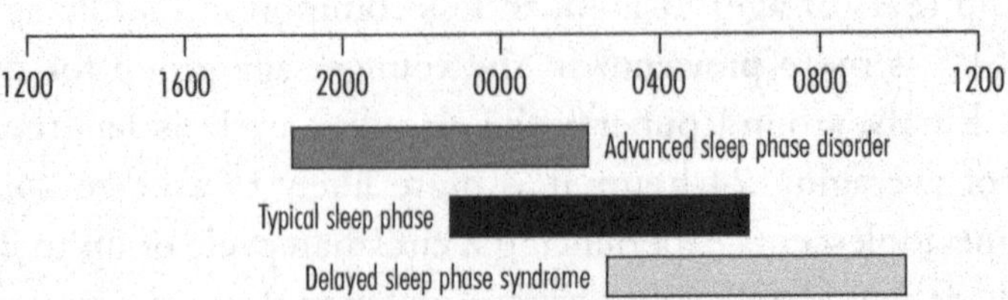

We saw with Josh's story in Chapter 10 the steps we need to follow if we have ASPS, so if you think this is you, and you have confirmed this by completing your alertness cycle, then go back, reread that chapter and follow those steps closely.

If you have confirmed you have DSPS by doing your cycle of alertness then follow the steps below, which aim to align our sleep with the environmental light/dark cycle.

Step 1: Assess your day

As with all the other sleep problems we have already discussed it is important to ensure that we firstly deal with the stresses of the day. This idea was discussed in detail in Chapter 8 so you can go back and reread it to refresh your memory.

Step 2: Understand the sleep process

If we suffer from DSPS treatment is simply a matter of trying to realign our circadian cycle of alertness with the more typical pattern – and the one that works better if we have the imperative of getting up before 9 am. Fortunately, when we are able to do this most of us will be able to sleep very well as there is nothing intrinsically wrong with our sleep. By understanding that the problem is simply one of timing we are much more likely to be diligent about the next step. Before you move to the next step though you might want to go back and reread Chapter 3 to reacquaint yourself with how sleep works because it is fundamentally important for anyone with DSPS to understand exactly what the sleep process involves.

Step 3: Moving your body clock – bright light therapy

One of the best aids for realigning our body clock is the use of bright lights.

When we are jet-lagged we implement this step without even thinking about it. Jet lag occurs as a consequence of flying across many time zones in rapid time. Frequently it means that in our new destination we either feel like sleeping very early in the evening and then being wide awake in the early morning hours, or we are wide awake at midnight, not feeling at all tired, until the early hours of the morning. In the first situation we have phase advanced (travelled east) and in the latter we have phase delayed (travelled west).

Regardless of whether we have phase delayed or phase advanced jet lag the quickest way we can achieve a realignment with our new destination is to fit in with the daily sleep–wake cycle at our new destination. Specifically people with jet lag are advised to:

1. Get exposure to bright lights in the early morning at your new destination.
2. Exercise in the late afternoon in the new time zone.
3. Eat at the time appropriate to your current location.
4. Minimise exposure to light (and computers etc.) in the evening.

Someone suffering from DSPS is in effect in permanent jet lag and often suffering from the same symptoms: headache, fatigue, fogginess and inability to sleep at the right time. It stands to reason therefore that if we apply the same rationale to resetting the body clock in DSPS as we do in jet lag then we will be highly likely to be successful.

So how do we do this when we are not actually changing time zones? The trick is bright light exposure at the *appropriate* time. If you have DSPS then you will need to be diligent in sticking to the following steps – but if you do, and maintain good sleep practices (Step 4) then you should be able to fall asleep at a normal hour and get the good, consolidated sleep you want.

Before starting the process of advancing the body clock you need to ensure you have chosen a time that allows you to be flexible as to the time you start your day. Ideally the process should be undertaken during a week or two of holidays. This is because, for the body clock to be successfully brought forward, you need to start the process at your preferred wake-up time, which is much later than normally required. For Charlotte, the most appropriate time was her school holidays.

1. Charlotte needed to work out her natural waking time. This was not the time that she *had* to get up every morning, but rather the time that she would naturally awake as when she was on holidays. Charlotte was already fairly aware of this time and knew that she would normally wake around 10.30 am whenever she hadn't been made to wake up earlier and so she used this time as her starting point.
2. For the next week Charlotte got up 30 minutes earlier each day. So day 1 she got up at 10.00 am; day 2 at 9.30 am; day 3 at 9.00 am; day 4 at 8.30 am and so on until day 7 when she got

up at the time she *had* to get up each day (7.00 am). To ensure she did wake up 30 minutes earlier each day she used an alarm. Every morning when the alarm sounded Charlotte would get out of bed and head for some bright sunshine and eat breakfast outdoors. She didn't wear sunglasses as this would have minimised the effect of the bright light.

3. Since it is known that exercise in the late afternoon will assist in advancing melatonin secretion, every afternoon around 5 pm Charlotte would do some form of exercise. As she enjoyed the gym this was not difficult. In the past she had often exercised in the morning but now she made a point of doing it in the late afternoon to maximise the potential for advancing her body clock. She took care though to complete her exercise by 6.30 pm as this ensured that the hormones produced during exercise, like cortisol, were not still active in her body when she went to sleep.
4. As the week wore on Charlotte found herself feeling a bit sleepier earlier in the evening and felt like she wanted to go to sleep just a little bit earlier, which she did. If she was not asleep within 30 minutes she got out of bed and waited until she felt sleepy again before trying to sleep.
5. For the next week or so Charlotte was vigilant with her 7 am wake-up time, exposure to morning sunshine and afternoon exercise and gradually her inclination to sleep came earlier and earlier so that by the end of the 2-week period she was falling asleep naturally around 11 pm.
6. A word of advice: it is important to consider the source of early morning light. While Charlotte was lucky and lived in an area where there was lots of sunshine, many of us do not, and often in the winter months sunshine is hard to find. In this case it is worthwhile investing in a bright light therapy device. Such devices are available on the internet and are proven to be as effective as sunlight, although undoubtedly not as much fun.

Step 4: Good sleep practices

Good sleep practices are fundamental to getting consolidated sleep whether or not you are a good or bad sleeper. In Charlotte's circumstances her body clock was clearly vulnerable to being shifted so anything that inadvertently delayed her body clock – as in exposure to bright lights at night (such as with a computer screen) – could set her clock back again. This meant that Charlotte had to closely watch her evening activities, make sure her exposure to light in the night-time was restricted and maintain a regular wake-up time.

Step 5: The use of melatonin

By choosing to follow steps 1–4 above and by maintaining a strict adherence to a sleep–wake schedule along with good sleep practices, Charlotte was able to maintain her normalised sleep–wake cycle. Sometimes, however, these modifications alone do not result in sufficient improvement and in these cases it may be that administration of melatonin may help advance the body clock.

In Australia, melatonin is available under prescription and should be taken only under a physician's advice. It is an addition to the steps outlined above – which must be followed if the phase delay is to be normalised.

The timing of melatonin is critical because if it is given at the wrong time it will further exacerbate the phase delay. In cases of DSPS, melatonin needs to be taken about 5–6 hours before the planned bedtime. In Charlotte's case, if she had required melatonin she would have taken it at 8 pm as her normal going-to-bed time was around 1 am. As the wake-up time is advanced each morning so too should the time that the melatonin is taken. So on the second evening, Charlotte would have taken the melatonin at 7.30 pm and so on until such time that the target bedtime is reached. For Charlotte, her bedtime target was 11 pm (as she had to get up at 7 am and she needed 8 hours' sleep) and so the gradual target for melatonin administration should be 6 pm. When the target time of 6 pm is reached, melatonin should be continued for another week and then discontinued.

In this chapter we have looked at a few of the more common sleep disorders that over the years may have caused us to have problems either getting to sleep, maintaining sleep or waking too early. We have discussed how to diagnose and treat these disorders and, because it is common to have more than one sleep problem, we have spoken about the steps to follow if we have any one, or a combination, of these disorders. Keep in mind though, that in this chapter and the next we discuss only the most prevalent sleep disorders. If you think you have a disorder causing your sleeplessness that has not been discussed it is important that you talk with your doctor. The sooner you find out about it the quicker you will be on your way to deep, restful sleep.

Chapter 12

Sleep apnoea

IF YOU HAVE SLEEP APNOEA and don't know it, chances are that you have trouble getting to sleep, or trouble maintaining sleep, or trouble staying asleep in the early morning hours, or any combination of these. This is because even though only about 10% of people who complain of sleeplessness have sleep apnoea, the majority of people with sleep apnoea (more than 60%) actually have insomnia symptoms.

Sleep apnoea, or as it is more correctly termed Obstructive Sleep Apnoea (OSA), is a relatively common disorder but it is largely undiagnosed. This is surprising because sleep apnoea is accompanied by the most obvious of signs – loud snoring. While snoring may be irritating to those who have to sleep nearby and may cause the person's partner to have sleepless nights, in most cases the snorer is blissfully unaware of the noise they are creating and in most cases it is not dangerous. It is important, however, to realise that snoring is the signature mark of sleep apnoea, especially if the snoring is accompanied by episodes of non-breathing and gasping.

Sleep apnoea affects about one in every twenty men and about one in every fifty women and the prevalence increases with age. Although sleep apnoea has been recognised for more than 100 years it is only in the last 30 years that its serious health effects have become clear. Before we discuss what these effects are we need to understand what causes sleep apnoea and then perhaps the reason why it is associated with so many other health problems will become apparent.

What is sleep apnoea?

When we breathe in through our nose (or mouth) the air has to pass firstly through our upper airway and then through our lower airway before eventually reaching our lungs. Our upper airway joins our lower airway at the trachea. If you feel along the front of the neck you will feel the cartilage rings of the trachea which protect this part of our airway from collapse. By contrast to the trachea, the upper airway, which is made up of mostly soft tissue, is susceptible to collapse under certain circumstances.

To understand why there is this susceptibility, we can think of our upper airway as similar to a water hose. The purpose of the hose is to deliver water from the tap to the bucket. Hoses generally work well provided we do not apply some form of external pressure that prevents the water from flowing. If we only squeeze the hose with a small amount of effort then the hose will partially close off and a small amount of water will continue to get through; however if, by applying a lot of effort, we manage to squeeze the hose totally closed then no water at all will get through until we release that pressure. How much pressure we need to apply to close off the hose depends upon the quality of the hose, or the age of the hose.

If we keep in mind this analogy of how the hose works we can begin to understand what happens to the upper airway during sleep to cause it to collapse.

When we are awake we are able to keep enough rigidity in the muscles of our upper airway to keep the airway open (like the hose) which is a good thing because it allows for the free passage of air from nose to lungs. When we sleep, however, all the muscles of the body relax, including the muscles of the upper airway. For most of us this is unproblematic and our muscles manage to maintain enough tension to keep the upper airway open, and as a result air flows freely through to our lungs. This uninterrupted flow of air is depicted in the following diagram.

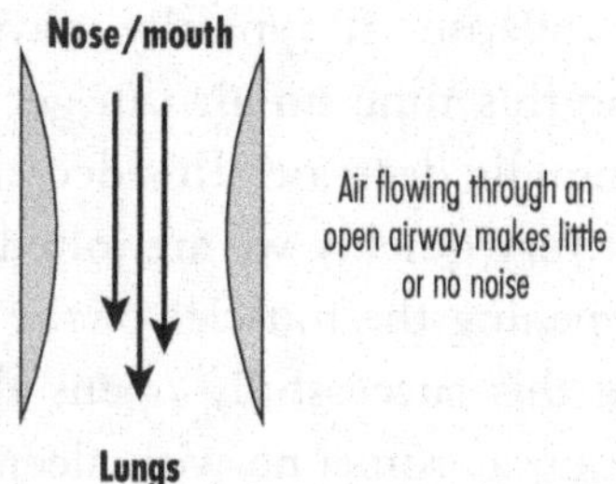

For those of us with sleep apnoea, however, our muscles lose too much tone when we go to sleep and become *too* floppy, such that when a small amount of pressure is applied (even just the force of gravity when we lie on our back) our airway, like the hose, begins to narrow and the air that gets through to our lungs is reduced (like the water in the narrowed hose). While the airway remains partially open, the airflow across the soft muscle tissue causes a vibration and it is this that is responsible for the telltale noise of snoring.

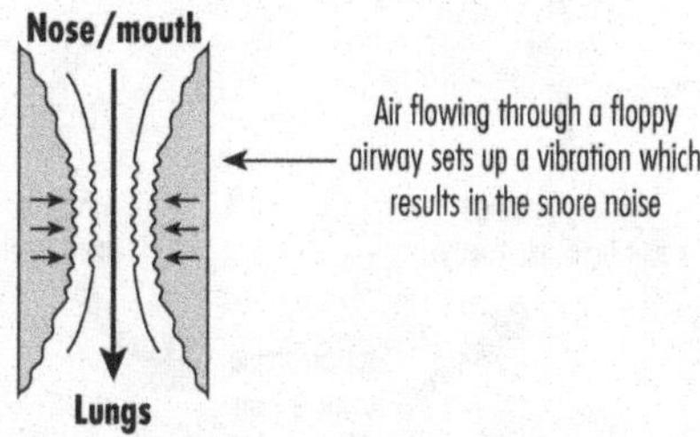

Once the airway starts to narrow and vibrate it is susceptible to total collapse. When the airway closes off completely, no air (like no water in the hose) can get through to the lungs. At this point there is no snoring because there is no airflow and this is referred to as an apnoea (from the Greek *a*, meaning without, and *pnous*, meaning breath).

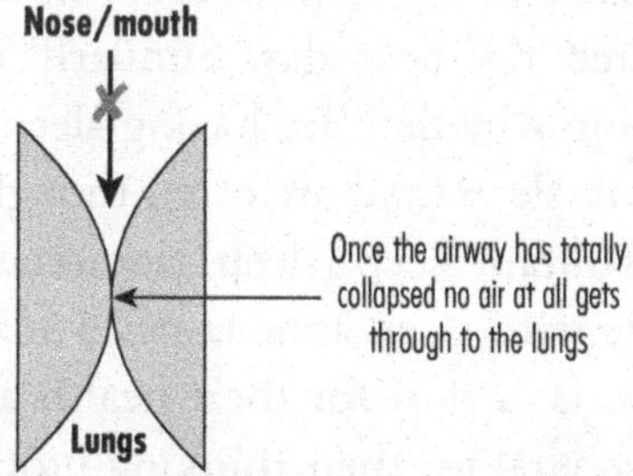

Once the airway collapses it typically stays closed for between 10–40 seconds. During this time no air can get to the lungs and our oxygen level starts to rapidly decrease. This decrease in oxygen is registered in our brain and very quickly we are jolted out of our sleep into wakefulness, thereby opening the muscles of the airway to let air back into our lungs. While this successfully opens the airway and allows air into the lung, as soon as someone with sleep apnoea goes back to sleep (usually within seconds) their airway will again begin to narrow, they will again start to snore and before very long (probably within about five snores) their airway will collapse again, only for the whole cycle to repeat itself over and over again throughout the sleep period. Someone with severe sleep apnoea will stop breathing more than 30 times an hour. If anyone has ever listened to someone with sleep apnoea this cyclical pattern of breathing will be familiar:

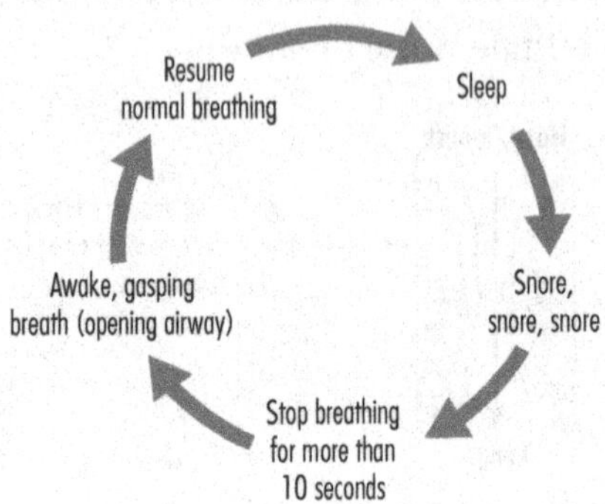

As a result of this ongoing cycle there is a constant disruption of sleep so that people with sleep apnoea are very sleep deprived and often suffer from extreme daytime fatigue. Because the awakenings do not last very long though, the majority of sleep apnoea sufferers are unaware that they wake up more than 30 times every hour and so have no idea why they are so tired the next day. Similarly many sufferers, again without understanding why they are having sleep problems, will find it difficult both to get to sleep (and are often thought to have sleep-onset insomnia) and to maintain sleep (sleep-maintenance insomnia). Additionally many people with sleep apnoea never manage to get the deep, restorative sleep that is critical for their health and well-being, or the REM sleep that is so vital for their thinking processes.

Sleep apnoea not only causes incredible disruption to our sleep but also longer-lasting health concerns. When we stop breathing we stop sending oxygen around our body and to all our cells that are so dependent on it. It is this deprivation of oxygen over and over again during our sleep, combined with the lack of sleep (due to the constant arousals), that result in the serious health consequences of sleep apnoea. We now know that if we have sleep apnoea and choose to do nothing about it we are much more likely to develop high blood pressure or have a heart attack or stroke. We also have a much higher risk of developing a metabolic disorder, such as type 2 diabetes or obesity, and more likely to have problems coping with the vagaries of life.

As if all this were not enough, a longitudinal study has shown conclusively that sleep apnoea is also associated with earlier death. In this study participants were assessed at baseline for sleep apnoea and were then followed for 18 years. At the end of this period an analysis of who had died over that time period was made. It was found that the vast majority of people without sleep apnoea (93%) were still alive, but almost one in two of those who had severe sleep apnoea at the start of the study (and chose not to treat it) had died.

Rick's story

Rick was 54 years old and his life was not going as expected. He had been prescribed antidepressants because he was finding it hard to cope, but he didn't think they were very effective as he still was having significant difficulty getting a good night's sleep.

His work had not been going well for a while and for the last few years he had felt like he had been in a state of disorganisation, constantly having difficulty remembering things and failing to follow up on some important issues. As it stood now, he had lost a lot of the motivation he used to have towards his work.

His personal life was also not going so well. He was newly single and when he talked about his separation, he recognised that he had probably become difficult to live with and was often angry at someone. He thought that the pressures of his working life had impacted in a big way on his relationship. This caused him a lot of stress, he started putting on weight, stopped exercising and bit by bit he lost interest in sex, which had really affected his ex-partner. In fact, while he did not want to talk about it, Rick was impotent – and this was also causing him a lot of anxiety.

Rick thought he might be a snorer. His ex-partner had mentioned that he snored, but that was some time ago, and since he and his ex-partner had had separate bedrooms for quite some time, he could not be sure. Certainly no one else had ever mentioned it. Rick was finding it increasingly difficult to get to sleep and, even when he managed to get to sleep fairly quickly, he would wake up many times, very hot and agitated and take up to about 30 minutes to get back to sleep. He admitted that he drank quite a bit at night when he was on his own as this seemed to relieve his sadness. He was, however, thinking about cutting back on this as he thought it was causing him to get up numerous times throughout the night to go to the toilet. He also suffered terrible heartburn which on some nights prevented him from getting almost any sleep.

Rick knew he had problems but didn't know what to do next.

Rick's story is more common than we would like to think. Rick presented to the doctor with a whole raft of problems, both professional and personal, and his initial presenting problem was having trouble maintaining sleep. Given that he had, by his own admission, a lot of home and work issues as well, it was not surprising that he would be diagnosed with, and be treated for, depression. However, as we have learned, sleep-maintenance insomnia and depression are often just the *symptoms* and not the actual problem. As Rick found, because the *cause* of his problem was not being treated he continued to suffer all the symptoms that were greatly affecting his ability to cope with life.

Fortunately, while waiting to see his doctor one day, Rick noticed a pamphlet which described sleep apnoea and some of the risk factors. When he talked to his doctor about this and mentioned that he had all the risk factors mentioned in the pamphlet, diagnosis followed fairly quickly.

Once treated, Rick was able to get his life slowly back in order. For a while, however, he was quite angry that it had taken so long to diagnose sleep apnoea – Rick thought that he had probably had this snoring problem for at least 5 years and nobody had even mentioned the possibility of him having something like this.

Unfortunately many people are not as lucky as Rick because, despite sleep apnoea's devastating effects on sufferers' health and quality of life, it remains largely undiagnosed. It is estimated that most people with sleep apnoea are unaware they have it, notwithstanding that mostly they are loud snorers.

So, how do we know if we might have sleep apnoea?

Apart from the telltale snoring there are a few other symptoms that we can look for, including pauses in breathing when sleeping, waking up gasping for air, morning headaches, daytime sleepiness, restless sleep, heavy sweating and frequent need to go to the toilet during the night. If you think that you or your partner may have sleep apnoea it is important that you do something about it because treating it will allow you to have uninterrupted sleep and improve your overall health and longevity.

While sleep apnoea can only be diagnosed by an overnight sleep study there are some predisposing factors which would make it more likely for you to have, or to develop, sleep apnoea. So if you snore and can tick any one (or more) of the boxes below then you should discuss the possibility of sleep apnoea with your doctor.

1. Overweight/obese ☐
2. Male ☐
3. Over 40 ☐
4. Family history of snoring ☐
5. Regular alcohol or sedative use ☐

As Rick was able to tick all the above boxes he was alerted immediately to the fact that sleep apnoea could be the cause of so many of his health and well-being issues.

Treatments

Today there are a variety of methods that can effectively treat sleep apnoea. The best method to use depends on a balance between the severity of the disorder, what is causing the disorder and patient choice, so it is best discussed with your doctor. There is a lot of information on available treatments and if you think you may have this disorder then it would be worthwhile taking time to research it.

The most common treatment for sleep apnoea is Continuous Positive Airway Pressure (CPAP) and this was what Rick chose. With this treatment, positive air pressure is delivered to the upper airway by means of a mask over the nose (or nose and mouth). This air pressure keeps the airway open and prevents the muscles from collapsing during sleep, allowing the person to breathe normally throughout the night. This stops the sleep disruptions and dips in oxygen, along with the subsequent adverse health effects, leaving the person feeling more energetic and alive than they have in years.

While CPAP treatment has been around for many years, and is the most popular therapy for sleep apnoea, a range of oral devices have recently been developed prevent the airway from collapsing and can be worn during sleep. These devices tend to work very well with mild sleep apnoea and are fitted by a dentist.

For some, the diagnosis and treatment of their sleep apnoea immediately resolves their problems with sleeplessness. Once they are able to breathe throughout the night they resume a normal pattern of sleep – undoubtedly getting the best sleep they have had in years. But this is not the case for everyone and certainly wasn't the case for Rick.

Rick and others like him have had sleep apnoea for a long time prior to a diagnosis. They have endured poor sleep for years and many, if not all, have developed bad sleep habits as well as a negative attitude towards their ability to sleep. This means that sometimes initiating therapy is just the start of the journey back to good sleep. Like the other people we have encountered in this book what is required is a systematic approach to the reclaiming of our deep, restful sleep.

There are a few steps we may need to follow, even after we commence therapy for our sleep apnoea.

Step 1: Assess your day

I have mentioned this step in many chapters – and it is often the one that is most overlooked. Always remember that how we spend our day may determine how we spend our night. So, if we have had a day full of challenges and have not adequately dealt with the stresses they have caused then we are likely to suffer the consequences of sleeplessness that night. In Rick's case he had a lot of daytime stress and so he needed to start doing all those things we have mentioned previously, like walking home from work and writing in a worry diary. Rick was somewhat surprised when he noticed what a difference just these small changes made.

Step 2: Understand the sleep process

If we understand the problems with our sleep process and the effect of sleep apnoea on our health and well-being we will realise that it is not because we are finding life difficult that we are finding sleep difficult but rather the reverse – it is because our sleep is so problematic that we suffer all the health and mood issues we saw in Rick. Once we know this we are much more likely to be diligent about the next step. If though, after reading this chapter (and perhaps even rereading Chapter 3), you are still finding it hard to understand the physiology of sleep apnoea it is important that you speak to your doctor about it.

Step 3: Maintain therapy

Often, when we start to feel much better physically and mentally, we forget just how bad we used to feel. At this stage, we are at risk of not being as diligent in maintaining our therapy and when this happens we will start to again suffer all the ill-consequences that we did before.

It is important to realise that therapy for sleep apnoea does not cure the disorder. The treatment is aimed at preventing the collapse of the upper airway during sleep. This means it needs to be used every night. This may seem incredibly obvious, but it is something that is often overlooked and many people use their therapy less and less, gradually feeling the worse for it. They usually then go back to the therapy, become diligent for a while and then the whole cycle starts over again. When we do this, we are creating all the negative effects of sleep apnoea and our see-sawing between therapy and non-therapy can do a lot of harm – both physically and mentally.

So far better that we make the effort to stick to the therapy as we will not only be well-slept but will be healthier and happier while living a longer life.

Step 4: Good sleep practices

As we have mentioned several times before, good sleep practices are fundamental to getting consolidated sleep and they are discussed in detail in Chapter 15.

For the moment though it is interesting to consider Rick's situation and see what he had to do in order for him to sleep well.

Firstly, Rick had to realise that alcohol was sabotaging his sleep – but not for the reasons he thought. Rick believed the volume of liquid he was drinking was causing him to go to the toilet a number of times during the night and this was the reason he was having such disrupted sleep. Actually, alcohol was sabotaging his sleep but it was doing so because it is a stimulant and after its initial sedative effect wears off (after 4–5 hours) its stimulating effects make sustaining sleep almost impossible. Rick's multiple trips to the toilet were the result not of the volume of liquid, but rather, a fairly common side-effect of sleep apnoea.

Secondly, Rick had to manage his heartburn which often made it difficult for him to get to sleep. While he thought that his heartburn may have been a consequence of eating too big a meal, he often had heartburn even if he didn't eat up big. As a result Rick had not bothered to modify his eating habits. What Rick failed to realise was that it was both his sleep apnoea and large meals that were causing the heartburn – and both things had to improve if he was not to be troubled by it. Along with increased need to go to the toilet during the night another telltale side-effect of sleep apnoea is heartburn, or as it is more correctly termed, gastro-oesophageal reflux. Once Rick's sleep apnoea was being well treated by his CPAP therapy and he stopped eating a big meal at night his heartburn improved.

Step 5: Practise CBT

Throughout this book we have talked about the importance of a positive attitude and how CBT can help us develop positive thinking. When we have sleeplessness for any period of time we cannot help but develop a negative attitude to our sleep, so CBT is an important part of getting our sleep back on track.

In Rick's situation the importance of CBT cannot be overemphasised. Rick chose CPAP therapy for his sleep apnoea because it is the most widely used treatment, but it does have downsides. It is sometimes difficult to start or stick with CPAP therapy. This can be for all sorts of reasons, but often it has to do with self-image and self-confidence. There would be few amongst us that would be overjoyed by the idea that whenever we sleep we need to wear a mask – which is exactly what Rick had to come to terms with. If Rick was going to succeed he needed to overcome his negative attitude towards the therapy, because as he had learned, his negative attitude led to negative thoughts which then caused a stress response which made sleep impossible, even if his apnoea was being treated.

For Rick, overcoming his negative attitude was not easy. His self-confidence and self-image was already suffering as his relationship had failed and he was impotent – and he definitely thought wearing a mask to bed would only add to his woes. Indeed whenever he thought about this he could feel himself becoming hot and agitated – a sure sign of the stress response.

What Rick had to come to terms with, and become positive about, was that his sleep apnoea was not him. It was a disorder and, while it caused a myriad of problems, it was treatable, and once treated he would live a normal, happy life. So instead of negative thoughts such as 'I look really unsexy with this mask'; 'women are going to laugh at me if they see me wearing this'; 'this mask makes me look as if I am on my deathbed', which made him feel very anxious, he was encouraged to think about the therapy more positively: 'Far better that my partner knows I care about my health'; 'This way my partner can sleep next to me because my snoring no longer drives her out of bed into the next bedroom'; 'I am a much nicer person when I sleep well so my partner will love me even more'; 'By wearing this mask I will sleep better and will be more productive at work and maybe get a promotion'. When Rick was able to develop these more positive thoughts he came to terms with his therapy and began to see it as a positive in his life rather than a negative. Certainly Rick would be the first to say that his life improved substantially once he began sleeping well.

It would be fair to say that Rick's story and his journey back to the land of good sleep may be familiar to many of us who have been diagnosed with sleep apnoea. While we may hope that the diagnosis and the treatment of the disorder is the total solution, it often isn't. It is the lucky ones amongst us who have no other problems to resolve before getting the sleep that we yearn for so much. Rick had to learn to adapt to the therapy, overcome some bad sleep habits, and come to terms with, and resolve, many of the anxious feelings he had for several years associated with sleep. Once he did this, which took about 4–5 weeks, Rick was able to sleep through the night, mostly undisturbed. On those nights he did wake to go to the bathroom he was able to fall back to sleep quite easily.

The other unexpected bonus for Rick, as it is for many people, was that he was once again able to be sexually active because he was no longer impotent. It is a sad fact, and one often not mentioned, that up to two-thirds of men with sleep apnoea have erectile dysfunction and that if the sleep apnoea is treated there is a significant improvement in sexual function; the more severe the sleep apnoea, the more the improvement upon therapy. This improvement in libido is also observed in women who suffer sleep apnoea. Women with sleep apnoea score much lower on the Female Sexual Function Index (FSFI) than women without sleep apnoea. Although no study has been published to date to show whether women's FSFI score improves with therapy there is no reason to think otherwise.

So, apart from the wonderful fact that treating sleep apnoea allows us to sleep well, feel well and be well it also helps us keep our relationships on track – for all sorts of expected and unexpected reasons.

Unlike other sleep disorders the treatment of sleep apnoea requires ongoing treatment and whether the therapy chosen is an oral appliance or a CPAP mask it needs to be used every night all night to have optimal efficacy. For this reason some of us will feel, like Rick, a little overwhelmed by a diagnosis and have been ignoring our snoring for years, not realising that it is at the heart of our fatigue and sleeping difficulties. Far from being overwhelmed though, we should consider a diagnosis of sleep apnoea a positive step forward in our quest for good sleep because it means that within a short period of time (and sometimes with a little bit of work) we will be getting that deep and restful sleep we have longed for. So don't put it off any longer – if you have been told you snore and feel tired and unmotivated a lot of the time, take the time to discuss this with your doctor. Renewed enthusiasm for living and a joyous vitality may just be your reward.

Chapter 13

Drugs and alcohol

WHILE IT PROBABLY COMES AS no surprise to most of us that there are many drugs that affect our ability to sleep, it may be a little more surprising to find that the drug most responsible for stealing our sleep is alcohol.

Alcohol

Alcohol plays a major role in nearly 10% of sleep troubles.

We have already mentioned that alcohol is not recommended as part of a good sleep practice. This is because, although it has an initial sedating effect, this is quickly dissipated and what ensues is a period of fragmented and disturbed sleep. For some of us, like Josh, alcohol use can creep gradually into our lives so that we don't recognise it as a problem. Sometimes, even when we're told this fact, we are reluctant to take it on board. It is common for us to consider our alcohol intake in terms of whether we are, or are not, a problem drinker. If we just like to drink at night, most nights, and we can choose to stop drinking whenever we wish, we will fall outside our definition of what we think of as a problem drinker and then proceed to assume that our drinking is harmless.

When we consider alcohol consumption in this way we focus mostly on how other people view our drinking in terms of our behaviour, or in other words, the social consequences (alcohol causing issues with relationships or work). We would be far better off, however, focusing on how alcohol affects us personally rather than socially, because the adverse physiological consequences when it comes to our sleep can be substantial.

Alcohol is a widely available and socially acceptable drug. Low levels of drinking often make us feel happy and have frequently been associated with a number of positive health effects. For example, a small amount of red wine has been linked with decreased cardiovascular risks. Alcohol is also, however, frequently overused and both moderate drinking (2 standard glasses of alcohol daily) and heavy drinking (3 or more glasses daily) have long been associated with adverse health outcomes. It has also been clear for quite some time that alcohol has a negative impact on our ability to have consolidated sleep.

Bill's story

Bill was 50 years old and had worked in the financial industry for most of his life. While it had always been quite stressful work he had enjoyed it and had been, and was, very successful. In the last few years, however, there had been a lot of uncertainty in his industry and his job had taken on a whole new level of stress. Bill was often feeling very anxious about where it was all going.

When the general downturn in economy first started he found, for almost the first time in his life, getting to sleep and staying asleep very difficult. He knew he was not able to quieten his brain sufficiently to allow sleep – and he would lie in bed at night thinking about all the possibilities of the financial world crashing around him. He would toss and turn throughout the night, seemingly drifting in and out of light sleep. He generally awoke feeling totally unrefreshed and exhausted and he found it increasingly difficult to concentrate and to motivate himself to meet the new challenges that were being presented.

At this time Bill, who had always enjoyed a drink, but generally only on weekends and rarely to excess, found that having a drink after work seemed to soothe his mind and actually allowed him to get to sleep – which was an absolute relief. Very soon, Bill found that having just the one drink did not seem to bring on sleep as well as it had at first and so he started having two drinks. Before too long he found himself, as Josh had, drinking at least three drinks every night and sometimes he even drank the whole bottle of wine on his own.

As Bill's night-time consumption of alcohol increased, he found that while he could get to sleep each night at about 10.30 pm, he was sleeping badly. His pattern of sleep was either that he regularly woke around 3 am, at which time he would go to the toilet and return to bed, but find it impossible to go back to sleep because his mind was racing. On these nights, despite wanting to sleep, he would end up getting up around 4–4.30 am and doing some work, even though he was very tired. On other nights he would again wake around 3 am, go to the toilet and then would manage to get back to sleep but only fitfully, seemingly just drifting in and out of light sleep until it was time to get up.

On average Bill was getting about 5 hours of consolidated sleep a night and so was severely feeling all the negative effects of sleep deprivation. In an effort to overcome his extreme tiredness and improve his concentration, which had really started to fail him, Bill started drinking coffee, and a lot of it. Unknown to Bill, caffeine is a stimulant and sleep stealer, so it was only adding to his feelings of stress. By the end of the day Bill really started looking forward to his evening drink (or drinks). The only trouble was that he seemed to need more and more alcohol to bring on his feelings of relaxation which enabled him to sleep. Bill thought that perhaps this was due to his excessive coffee intake, and in one sense this was true. Certainly caffeine had a role to play in Bill's sleep difficulties, but a more primary problem was his alcohol intake.

While Bill had a long way to go before he became what we think of as a problem drinker, his drinking was certainly causing him problems biologically. Regrettably, his story is typical of many who struggle with sleep and is more common than we might think. It was only when Bill fully understood the effects of alcohol on sleep that he was finally able to break the cycle.

Naturally enough, at first Bill didn't really think giving up alcohol was a good idea – as he now relied upon it to fall sleep. He thought that a far better strategy would be to try hard to decrease his coffee intake and then perhaps have the occasional sleeping pill at night to allow him to sleep throughout the night.

Many people, when confronted with a sleep problem, try to self-medicate. Initially, this often involves alcohol, and then sleeping pills. Sleeping pills can be effective in alleviating sleeplessness and reducing fatigue, and they can be an important part of short-term treatment for someone who is having problems sleeping. It can also make sense to prescribe an antidepressant to someone who isn't sleeping as they will be in a negative mood state (depression) and a hallmark of depression is either early morning awakenings or waking after 4–5 hours of sleep.

While these prescription drugs may alleviate the problem in the short term they do not present long-term solutions. It is far more important that the person understands the processes of sleep and learns how to manage them effectively so that they can regularly get deep, restful sleep.

Rather than taking sleeping pills to assist him to maintain his sleep, Bill needed to understand that what he was doing was perpetuating his sleeping problem. As with all the other sleeping problems we have discussed, he also needed to follow some steps which would eventually allow him to sleep through the night undisturbed.

Step 1: Understand how alcohol interrupts the sleep cycle

Before we are prepared to make efforts to change, most of us need to know why the change is so necessary. Bill came to rely on his evening drinks, and even to enjoy them – and unless there was a good reason to stop this practice he was somewhat disinclined to do so. Bill needed to learn the physiological effects of alcohol on his body, and once he understood these he was far more prepared to reduce his alcohol intake.

1. While alcohol has an initial sedating effect, it is rapidly metabolised and after 4–5 hours there is minimal blood alcohol remaining (assuming a pre-sleep concentration of no more than

about 0.09%. How many drinks it takes to get to this blood alcohol level is highly dependent upon the weight of the person, but on average is somewhere between 3–5 drinks.) After this time the person experiences what is known as 'rebound wakefulness', which can mean periods of shallow sleep and multiple awakenings, sweating, increased heart rate and overall general activation (as opposed to the normal quietness associated with sleep). So rather than increasing sleep, alcohol actually causes a reduction in total sleep time.

2. Not only does alcohol affect the amount of sleep we have but it also affects our quality of sleep. Alcohol consumption actively suppresses REM sleep, which is so important to how well we think and feel the next day.
3. A tolerance to alcohol's sedating effects builds up quickly, so that within 5 nights an increase in alcohol consumption will be required to produce the same sleep-inducing effects.
4. Alcohol also causes a number of sleep disorders to worsen – restless legs, sleep apnoea – which, as we learned in the previous chapters, further reduces the quality and quantity of sleep.

Time and again, these effects of alcohol on sleep have been shown experimentally but, despite this, alcohol remains one of the most used sleep aids for those of us who, like Bill, experience difficulty getting to sleep.

Once Bill understood what alcohol did to his body, and why it caused such bad sleep, he was much more open to quitting his evening drinks. He still needed to unwind from the day, however, and by following Step 2 he learned other ways of relaxation.

Step 2: Assess your day

Previously, when we have discussed the other causes of secondary insomnia, I have always put this step first. In Bill's situation, however, and for others who suffer like him, cutting out alcohol is the most important step. Once that is accepted and taken on board, implementing these other steps will more easily follow. As we have discussed this step in other chapters I will only note here the things Bill started to do that he felt improved his sleep.

Bill started to assess his day and appropriately deal with any issues that had arisen during the day. Bill introduced some exercise into his routine and, because he was so busy at work and had no time, he started getting off the bus a stop early. Over time, he found himself getting off the bus earlier and earlier, gradually increasing his walking time. He also started keeping a worry diary, which worked well for him. On particularly stressful days he would get home, change out of his work clothes and do a relaxation exercise – he found the deep breathing exercise the most beneficial. Deep breathing (as described in Chapter 6) really seemed to calm him down and, because he felt much calmer after doing it, he found that he did not look for an alcoholic drink as soon as he got home. This was a defining change because he found that if he did not start drinking when he first got home, he found it easier not to drink for the rest of the night.

Step 3: Follow good sleep practices

Good sleep practices are discussed in detail in Chapter 15. These practices are essential for everyone to follow. Bill particularly needed to understand why coffee had the effect it did and cut back on it. He gradually decreased his caffeine consumption and stopped drinking coffee after lunch. He found that instead of relying on caffeine for his afternoon pick-me-ups he could do some exercise at that time – which was also effective in decreasing his level of tiredness.

Step 4: Practise CBT

As we have found in earlier chapters, CBT can be effective in many sleep problems. Mostly, when we have relied on something for a while to help us sleep, like alcohol or sleeping pills, we begin to believe that we will not be able to sleep without that aid. This is not the case as sleep is a natural process, and as long as we allow the natural processes to occur we will be able to sleep. What we have learned though, is that just thinking the thought 'I won't be able to get to sleep without drinking' will, of itself, cause us not to sleep. So we need to address this thought and turn it into a positive thought and behaviour.

With Bill, once he was in the position to contrast the difference between the adverse outcomes alcohol had on his sleep to the positive effects of exercise, practising relaxation and keeping a worry diary, he was able to use CBT to good effect. Instead of thinking 'If I don't have a few drinks I won't be able to get to sleep for hours', he was able to think more positive thoughts, like 'The less I drink the more I will sleep' or 'Being naturally relaxed will give me the best night of sleep'.

By following all of these steps Bill started to get the sleep he had been missing out on and for this he was very grateful. Although, since he did like the occasional drink, he was concerned that if he wanted good sleep he might not be able to drink again, ever. This is not the case. As Bill was somewhat relieved to discover, low consumption of alcohol – one beer (340 ml) or a glass of wine (150 ml) – causes little to no sleep disturbance. Any more than that has the capability to cause a substantial impact on the quality and quantity of sleep. For Bill, this meant that if in the future he wanted to have more than one drink he understood that his sleep would be impacted and that he would experience fatigue and a level of fogginess the next day. He was now well aware that drinking and sleeping do not make happy bedfellows and that to rely on alcohol to sleep only results in sabotaging sleep.

Drugs

Sometimes a person may turn not to alcohol but to drugs. Up to 5% of people with sleep problems will have a problem with using drugs inappropriately. Both illicit drugs and prescribed drugs are easily obtained and many of them will cause problems with our sleep. About 4% of sleeplessness is caused by substance use other than alcohol. While we may think it is mostly the illicit drugs causing these problems this is not borne out by research. There are now many prescribed drugs, either used as directed or abused, that cause sleep problems.

If you think you may have sleeplessness due to a drug you have been prescribed, it is important to discuss this matter with your doctor. You should see if there are any alternatives that you may take that will not have this particular effect on you, or whether, by taking the drug at another time of day, it will improve your sleep ability. Fortunately it is now a regulation in most countries that drug companies list all the potential adverse effects of a drug so we are usually able to discover if a drug we have been prescribed may be causing our sleeplessness.

This, however, is not the case for illicit drugs and most people take these without ever knowing what effect they have on either our health or sleep in the short or long term.

In Australia more than a third of the population have at some stage in their life used an illicit substance. Marijuana is the most common (used by about 30% of the population at some time in their lives) followed by amphetamines (10%), ecstasy or MDMA (8%), cocaine (5%) and heroin (1%).

'Wakeful' drugs

Being under the influence of any of the drugs mentioned above (with the exception of marijuana) will allow us to have prolonged periods of wakefulness – which is why they are used on the party scene. After the drug wears off though, the user will experience rebound sleepiness and over the next 48 hours will sleep more than usual (a bit like sleeping in on the weekends when we have not had enough sleep during the week). This may lull the user into a false sense of security thinking that, because the effects of the drug have worn off and they have caught up on their sleep, that their sleep is now back to normal (until perhaps the next time).

However, this is not the case and, for many people, once the rebound sleep has been had the subsequent sleep is anything but normal. Research now shows us that for a period of days, weeks or months (depending on usage and susceptibility) the sleep that ensues is characterised by persistent insomnia, prolonged sleep latency (or sleep-onset insomnia) and altered sleep structure.

The persistent insomnia, and particularly the difficulty getting to sleep, appears to be a common outcome for most of the psychoactive drugs but the change in sleep structure seems to be dependent on the type of drug taken. For example, with cocaine and amphetamine there is a sustained decrease in REM sleep; with heroin or morphine there is a sustained decrease in deep sleep; and with MDMA there is a sustained increase in very light, stage 1 sleep. This means that while the user has the short-term (and desired) effect of prolonged wakefulness counteracted in the short term by rebound sleepiness, they are at risk of developing significant long-term sleeplessness with all its subsequent negative health and well-being consequences.

Most people are unaware of the drugs' potential to cause persistent insomnia. This may in part be because there is always a delay between cause and effect. For example, if we were to take a tab of ecstasy on a Friday night, we would (depending on how much we took) stay awake for the next 24 hours at which point we would want to sleep much more than normal for the next 48 hours (our rebound sleep period). By the Monday night, and for some time thereafter, we may be finding it difficult to get to sleep. When we do sleep we might feel as if we are only drifting on the edge of sleep. It is unlikely though that we will make the connection between our sleeplessness and the drug-taking because the sleeplessness is suffered days after taking the drug, and we probably only ever thought the effects of the drug were short term.

The inability to make this important connection means that many people do not attribute their sleeplessness to their weekend drug-taking but view it as a separate, working-week issue, which may then lead to a misdiagnosis of anxiety, depression and perhaps a prescription for sleeping pills or antidepressants.

Unfortunately, unlike the other sleeping problems, if we have used any of these drugs and are having trouble sleeping it is difficult to improve sleep right away simply by following a set of steps. What is crucial is that we realise what is causing the sleeplessness and aim to stop using any of these drugs. Regaining good sleep will take time and is a matter of allowing the sleep pathways to be re-established naturally. In the meantime, it is important that you speak with your doctor about undertaking the necessary lifestyle changes. The steps set out for Bill earlier could improve sleep and make it easier to come by. Eventually deep, restful sleep will come.

Marijuana

In contrast to the 'wakeful' drugs we have spoken about above, marijuana is different because how it affects us is dependent on the dose we take. Marijuana has been used for thousands of years for its psychoactive and purported medicinal qualities, and today it is the most widely used illicit drug. It is frequently viewed as a benign drug but whether this is the case is dependent upon dose and usage. It can be classified in a number of ways such as a hallucinogen, a psychedelic, or as a drug that causes an altered state of consciousness with mild euphoria and relaxation. The active ingredient in marijuana is Tetrahydrocannabinol (THC). In low doses (4–20 mg THC) it is a mild sedative; in moderate doses (20–50 mg THC) a stimulant; and in large doses (more than 50 mg THC) a psychedelic, which may cause psychotic-like symptoms.

As with its effects on us, the effects of marijuana on our sleep will vary with how much is taken and the regularity of usage. Low doses decrease the amount of REM sleep, but increase both deep sleep and total sleep time. This sounds like good news for the troubled sleeper but disappointingly these increases gradually reduce to baseline levels after a week of nightly use. So while many people claim to use low doses of marijuana as a sedative, it actually loses its somewhat limited effect on aiding sleep within just one week, after which time there is a habituation to the drug.

In higher doses, although total sleep time does not appear affected, both REM sleep and deep sleep is decreased which, as we know, has significant health, cognitive and mood consequences. Discontinuation of marijuana in this higher dosage range also causes significant sleep symptoms for the majority of users (between 70–80%) with persistent sleep-onset insomnia as well as a significant decrease in REM sleep. If you are a regular moderate-to-heavy user of marijuana it is important that you know about these very real sleep disturbances because for some people they are so great that they cause them to relapse back to marijuana use in order to improve their sleep quality during a quit attempt.

Marijuana is vulnerable to abuse. Low doses appear to have no long-term effect on our sleep and, indeed after a limited time, do not even appear to have the sedative effect that some may believe. Research clearly shows that regular moderate-to-heavy use has a significant impact on our sleep.

If you are currently, or have been in the past, a regular user of marijuana (smoking it more than five times per week) it is likely that you have sleeping problems, especially if you are trying to quit the drug.

Marijuana may well be viewed as a benign drug but it, like alcohol, can have far-reaching effects on our sleep.

Sleeping pills

Drugs and alcohol have a significant and extended impact on the quality of our sleep when we are under their influence, but they also cause significant problems when we stop taking them. For this reason many of us will seek out other types of drugs, such as sleeping pills, to help us overcome these negative sleep effects, but this then brings its own set of problems.

Sleep medications can be useful in the short term and they play an important role in terminating the negative spiral of night after night of sleeplessness. They are one of the most widely used medications globally and while it is difficult to estimate usage it is thought that about 10% of adults use over-the-counter sleep aids and about 10% use prescription medications. In contrast to the past, the use of sleeping pills is no longer largely the domain of the elderly. Sleeplessness appears to be affecting individuals across all age groups and there has been a twofold increase in the use of sleeping aids by people in the 20–45 age group.

Thankfully today's newer types of sleeping pills (non-benzodiazepine hypnotics) do not carry the same risks of physical dependence and overdoses as previous pills and it is unlikely that physical dependence will occur. Psychological dependence on these pills as a consequence of long-term use, on the other hand, can still be powerful, and can leave people feeling convinced that they cannot get a good night's sleep without them. They become reluctant to stop using them and if they do stop they will frequently experience rebound insomnia (which is normally of short duration), which further reinforces the idea that they cannot sleep without the medication.

Like other drugs, sleeping pills change the structure of sleep. On the plus side, they normally decrease the time it takes to get to sleep and the number of nocturnal awakenings along with the total amount of sleep. However, they commonly increase the amount of time spent in light sleep (stages 1 and 2 NREM) and decrease the amount of time spent in REM and deep sleep – stages of sleep that we know are critically important for good thinking and good metabolic health. It is also the case that sleeping pills, like all medications, can have some unwanted side effects. Despite the improvement in the length of time the newer drugs stay in the system (reduced half-life) people can often experience grogginess upon wakening, daytime dizziness, nausea and increased appetite.

Sleeping pills may help you get some much-needed rest in the short term (2–4 weeks) but they are not the long-term answer.

The best approach is not to reach for the pill, but to address whatever is the underlying cause of your sleeplessness and deal with it.

So if you are trying to reduce your reliance on alcohol or drugs the best approach is not to swap one problem for another. Rather, try to improve your sleep by following some of the many suggestions in this book, like the steps recommended for Bill.

Dealing with sleep problems takes time, but with perseverance you will achieve deep, restful sleep.

Chapter 14

Primary insomnia

UP UNTIL NOW WE HAVE spent a lot of time discussing secondary insomnia. There is a good reason for this – most sleeplessness is the result of some other factor, and once this is identified and treated the insomnia will resolve. In contrast to this, primary insomnia, which affects about 12% of people with sleeping difficulties, will only be diagnosed once all other potential causes have been ruled out.

Primary insomnia may not occur alone, and in fact commonly presents in combination with secondary insomnia. Once the cause of the secondary insomnia is resolved (for example, once the sleep apnoea is treated) the primary insomnia will be unmasked, at which point it will need to be dealt with before all the sleep problems are resolved.

As in secondary insomnia, primary insomnia can cause disruptions in sleep at the start of the night (sleep-onset insomnia), during the night (sleep-maintenance insomnia) or at the end of the night (early-morning-awakening insomnia). Whatever shape it takes, primary insomnia has the same effect on us as secondary insomnia and we suffer all the same negative consequences of sleep deprivation that we have discussed.

So what are we really talking about when we say primary insomnia? There are a number of different types of primary insomnia, but we are going to discuss the three most common: psychophysiological insomnia or 'learned' insomnia, sleep state misperception, and insomnia due to poor sleep hygiene.

'Learned' insomnia

Frequently we deliberately disrupt our sleep processes when, for some reason, we do not want to sleep. Say for example, we have a major report due and the deadline is rapidly approaching. We have to work long days in order to finish the report and so to keep ourselves awake we drink lots of coffee until late in the night. When we do end up going to bed we find we cannot sleep due to the alerting effects of the caffeine. As most of us have experienced, this type of acute wakefulness comes to an end once the report is submitted and the caffeine intake is reduced.

This type of wakefulness is not so distressing as we know the reason for it and we can do something about it. Problems arise, however, when, due to bad sleep habits, we *unknowingly* disrupt the sleep processes turning what should be a brief bout of insomnia into something lasting weeks and maybe months. In these situations it is not unusual for the person to develop an alerting response to sleep, so that even when they rectify the bad sleep habit – say, drinking too much coffee – they still do not get the sleep they need as they have developed an over-concern about their inability to sleep. Simply put these people have 'learned' to worry about their sleeplessness. While this may appear to be a consequence of anxiety, people suffering from learned insomnia do not score highly on the anxiety scale in Chapter 5 and the core of their sleeplessness is their belief that they are bad sleepers.

Learned insomnia can present as any of the types of insomnia we have already discussed and many of the steps outlined in those chapters apply equally well here. If you think you may have learned insomnia it is important that you go back and read the chapter that applies to your type of sleeplessness, whether it be sleep onset, sleep maintenance or early morning awakening, and start following the steps outlined there. The following three steps are of particular importance to anyone with learned insomnia.

Step 1: Follow good sleep hygiene

Good sleep habits are particularly important for people with learned insomnia as research indicates that these people are particularly vulnerable to sleep disturbances. For example, an irregular bedtime may not be a problem for someone with robust sleep but it would cause sleeplessness for someone prone to learned insomnia.

The fact that our sleep may not be as robust as someone else's sometimes causes concern for those of us who suffer from learned insomnia and we begin to believe that we are not able to sleep like others. This is not the case. Just as some people are better runners or better thinkers, some people are better sleepers. That doesn't mean that you can't run or think or sleep – it just means that you might have to put more time and energy into developing the ability.

One way to do this is to pay special attention to your sleep habits (just as a runner who wants to improve their race results would pay special attention to their footwear). Good sleep habits are outlined in detail in the next chapter, so it is important that you pay special attention and start implementing them as soon as possible.

Step 2: Practise CBT

If you think you might have learned insomnia it is important that you understand exactly what CBT is and how it works because CBT has been shown to be highly effective in overcoming this. Learned insomnia occurs when a person *believes* they are a bad sleeper and that they will always, or nearly always, find sleep difficult. The reason why they come to believe this is normally unknown, although sometimes it can be traced back to a particular incident. More often than not the belief is of such long standing that how it came about is no longer relevant. What is relevant is the belief itself – and this is the very core of CBT. By addressing this belief and changing the thoughts around it we will be able to improve our sleep.

People suffering chronic learned insomnia will over the years have developed thought patterns that constantly sabotage their attempts to sleep. Thoughts such as:

- 'I am a really bad sleeper.'
- 'I will never be able to get to sleep.'

- 'Everyone else always sleeps well, why can't I?'
- 'I can't wake up during the night because that means I will not be able to get back to sleep again and I will be exhausted tomorrow.'
- 'I will lie awake all night, again!'

Thoughts like these only serve to increase anxiety and, because of the stress response, they make sleep even more elusive. People with learned insomnia are often aware of these negative thoughts but feel powerless to stop them, thereby almost guaranteeing that they will not get the sleep they desire. By implementing CBT we will be able to control these feelings and effectively stop the stress response, which will allow for good, consolidated sleep.

To practise how to do this let's look at the problems Patrick was having sleeping and how he overcame them.

Patrick's story

Patrick had been having trouble sleeping for most of his adult life and although he was nearly always diligent with his going-to-bed routine he was still unable to get good sleep. He did not have any particular worries in his life, and on the whole he felt relatively relaxed, but he just could not get good sleep. He frequently took a long time to get to sleep and found it difficult to get back to sleep if he woke during the night.

When asked about what he was thinking at these times he was vaguely aware that his mind was active with all sorts of jumbled thoughts, but he could not pinpoint anything in particular. Although it took him some time, Patrick was eventually able to map out what he thought was happening to him at night: when he went to bed at night, even though he was tired, he would begin to worry almost immediately about his ability to sleep – about whether he would fall asleep, whether he would stay asleep, or whether he would get enough sleep. He believed he thought this way because he had come to think of himself as a 'bad sleeper' who would always have trouble sleeping.

Once he was able to recognise this thought (or cognition) and understand that for him it was a negative thought, then he could start to break the whole process down. He began to see that worrying about whether he could sleep evoked the stress response, causing all the physical side effects of his heart rate increasing and his brain racing, which effectively prevented him from getting to sleep and left him tossing and turning for what seemed like half the night.

By putting this all down in a diagram (see below), Patrick was quickly able to see the interaction between his thoughts and behaviour and to understand what was happening to him on a nightly basis.

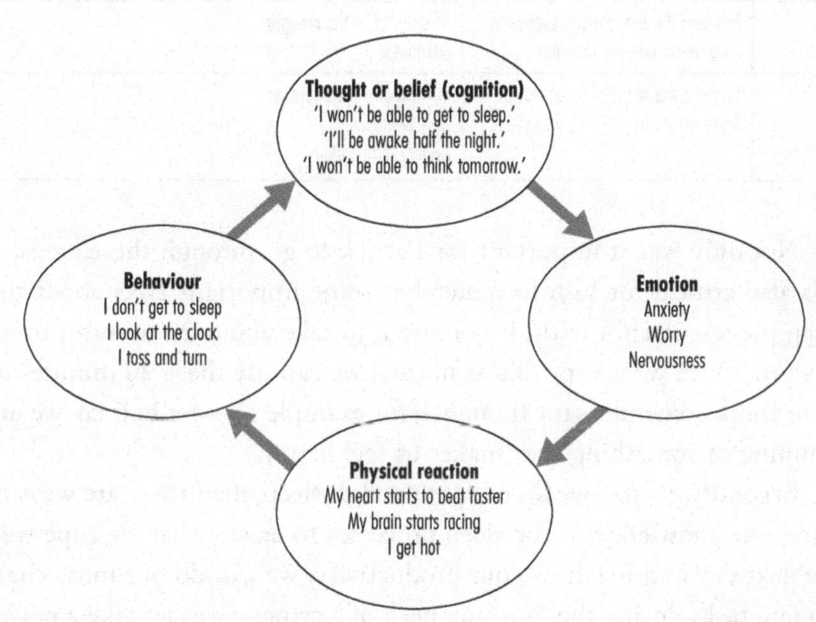

So, how did Patrick get in control of these thoughts? Patrick had to learn to deal with his negative night-time thoughts in the same way as people have to deal with their negative daytime thoughts. How he did this is outlined in the following table.

Step	Action	Patrick's situation
1	Recognise the trigger (or situation)	Turning out the light to go to sleep
2	Recognise the automatic thoughts (or cognitions)	'I am such a bad sleeper I won't be able to get to sleep for ages.' 'If I don't get to sleep quickly I won't get to sleep for ages and won't be able to think tomorrow.'
3	Recognise the emotional response to thoughts	Anxiety and nervousness
4	Evaluate physical response to emotions	Increased heart rate, brain racing, feeling hot
5	Consider alternate, more positive thoughts	'I haven't slept well many times before and I have managed quite well so far.' 'If I feel really tired during the day I can have a 15-minute power nap or go for a brisk walk in the sunshine, either of which will wake me up sufficiently to get through the afternoon.' 'Oh well, I always get to sleep eventually and I will tonight as well.'
6	Examine the emotional response to these more positive thoughts	Acceptance of the thought Calmness
7	Evaluate the physical response to these emotions	Release of muscle tension Easy breathing Normal temperature

Not only was it important for Patrick to go through these steps, it was also critical for him to remember some important facts about the sleep process itself. Firstly, it is normal to take about 20 minutes to go to sleep. Once we accept this as normal we can use these 20 minutes or so to think some pleasant thoughts, for example about a holiday we are planning or something that makes us feel happy.

Secondly, even if we do not get enough sleep, then there are ways of using our knowledge of the sleep processes to ensure that we cope well the next day and maximise our productivity: we can do our most challenging tasks during the morning peak of alertness; we can take a power nap of up to 20 minutes to decrease our sleepy chemicals and to refresh our thinking processes; and we can take a walk outside during the afternoon lull, which will stimulate our awake pathways. Once Patrick understood these things and put them into practice his worry about sleep decreased significantly and he managed to sleep much better on a regular basis. He actually came to understand that he was not a 'bad sleeper' but was indeed capable of very good sleep, and this realisation in itself improved his sleep. That is not to say Patrick never experienced poor sleep again – because this is surely not the normal human state. Since he had learned the skills to cope with the problem, however, he was able to manage these times well.

Successfully implementing CBT to break down our negative thought processes will take time and practice but it is well worthwhile persevering as it has been shown to be an effective tool in treating learned insomnia. This is especially so if we use our knowledge of our sleep processes, as Patrick was encouraged to do, to develop our alternate, more positive thoughts.

Step 3: Get out of bed if you do not fall asleep within 30 minutes of going to bed or after a nocturnal awakening

We have spoken about this before in chapters 8 and 9 so I will not go into too much detail here. This step is especially important for those of us who have learned insomnia because the longer we are awake in bed, the more it serves to confirm our belief that we are bad sleepers. This in turn initiates our stress response, which prolongs our wakefulness.

As we know, it is normal to take about 20 minutes to fall asleep and if we take longer than this we are either not tired enough to fall asleep or we are having trouble initiating sleep. In either case, the best thing we can do is get out of bed and wait until we feel sleepy again. If we don't do this we run the risk of lying in bed, awake, thinking all those negative thoughts such as 'I am never going to get to sleep', 'Why is sleep so hard' and we will produce more of the stress hormones that make sleep elusive.

When we get up we need to sit in a warm, dimly lit room and perhaps do some relaxation exercise or read a magazine, or even practise some CBT. Once we start to feel sleepy again (yawning, eyes drooping) we can go back to bed and go to sleep. If again we cannot fall asleep within a reasonable time then we need to get up again and continue to do so until we naturally fall to sleep. While doing this it is important just to approximate the time and not to clock-watch as this will more often than not promote a stress response – 'Oh no, it's already midnight and I am not asleep yet!' Instead, we need to use our innate knowledge of our selves to know when we no longer feel sleepy or inclined to sleep. It is at that point that we need to get out of bed and wait until we feel sleepy once more before we again attempt sleep.

For those of us with learned insomnia these three steps are of great importance and if we're diligent with them we should quickly see an improvement in our ability to get to sleep and to maintain sleep. Keep in mind that there are other strategies that pertain to sleep-onset (Chapter 8) and sleep-maintenance insomnia (Chapter 9) – so it may be worthwhile to revisit those chapters and follow all the steps set out there.

Sleep state misperception

This is also known as 'paradoxical insomnia' and we spoke about it briefly in Chapter 10. It occurs when a person thinks they are awake for a large part of the night, but in fact, it turns out that they have been asleep for most of the night. While this may seem impossible it is more common than we realise, especially in the early hours of the morning when we are in and out of our light sleep. While most of us, at various times, can experience sleep state misperception it is found more frequently in people who report insomnia.

If we consider once more our sleep profile we will begin to understand how this misperception can come about. In the early hours of the morning when we are more often in the lighter stages of sleep, sometimes brief awakenings occur within 30 to 45 minutes of each other. At these times, without realising it, we go back to sleep, probably fairly quickly. When we then wake up again 45 minutes later, and because we don't know that we have gone back to sleep in the first place, we think we have been awake the entire time. While this does not have to be a problem it can become one if we start to get anxious about our perceived lack of sleep because this will create a more permanent problem.

The following sleep profile diagram shows multiple awakenings in the early hours of the morning relatively close together (shaded area). When this occurs we begin to think that we were awake for a lot longer than we actually were. Indeed this sleep profile is an approximation of the sleep profile of Madeleine, a woman who had been having considerable trouble staying asleep in the early morning hours.

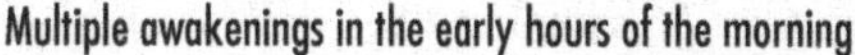

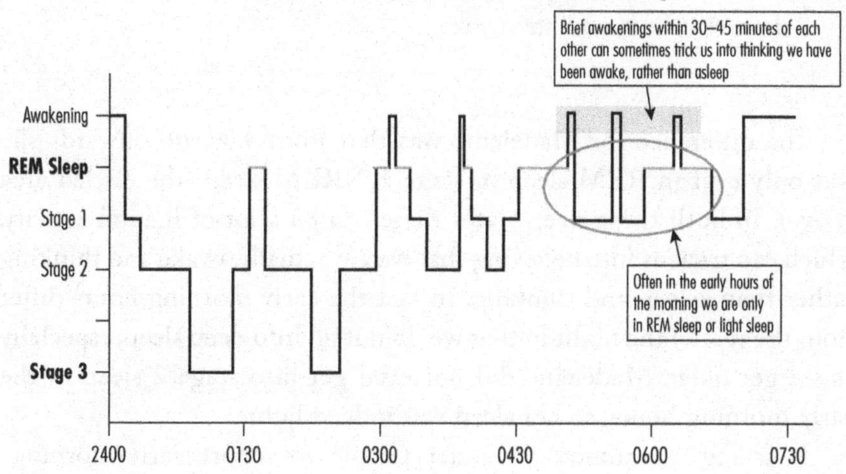

Madeleine's story

Madeleine is 56 years old and had always enjoyed being a late riser. She did not usually go to bed much before midnight as she enjoyed staying up a bit after all her family went to bed so that she could enjoy some quiet time. In the past this had worked well for her as she did not need to get up until about 8 am each morning. However for the past 6 months she had been having trouble staying asleep much past 4.30–5 am, which meant she was only averaging about 5–6 hours every night and, although she felt she was coping well with her lack of sleep her inability to sleep in the early morning was becoming very frustrating and she was now becoming anxious about her sleep.

Madeleine's doctor wondered whether she might be suffering from mild depression but Madeleine did not think this was the case and opted for a sleep study to see what might be going on. What she found out about her sleep really surprised her. From her sleep study and the sleep profile above she could see that she had woken around 4.30 am (as she did every morning) but she actually fell asleep again fairly quickly and mostly stayed asleep until she awoke at around 6.30 am with three periods of brief awakenings in between. So, unbeknownst to Madeleine, she had actually been mostly sleeping from 4.30 am and not awake.

The difference for Madeleine was that from 4.30 am onwards she was only ever in REM sleep or stage 1 NREM sleep (the circled area above). In both these sleep states there can be a lot of mental activity, which can trick us into believing that we are actually awake and thinking rather than asleep and thinking. In fact the early morning hours differ from the rest of the night in that we do not go into deep sleep, especially as we get older. Madeleine did not even get into stage 2 sleep in the early morning hours, so her sleep was indeed light.

It is fairly common for older people to report early-morning-awakening insomnia and while this is a very real problem for some, for others it is a case of sleep state misperception. For these people it is important that they understand what is going on to allay any anxiety about their sleep.

One easy way of detecting whether we have been awake or asleep is to think about what has gone on during the 'awake' period. If we think we have been lying awake we need to try to remember what we have been thinking about. If we can't remember very much then it is more likely than not that we have actually been asleep. We might remember little snippets of information, which probably indicates that we were in light sleep; or we might remember a bizarre dream-like experience, which is indicative of coming out of REM sleep – either way we were asleep and not awake for the period of time we thought we were. It is important to do this quick check as it can have a big impact on how we view our sleep time.

If we think our early morning wakefulness may be due to sleep state misperception, and if it continues to cause us concern, we could try using an Actigraph. This is a wristwatch type of device that detects movement. When we are asleep we do not move very much, but when we lie in bed awake our movements increase. By measuring the difference in our level of movement the Actigraph is an easy and fairly accurate way to establish whether we are awake or asleep in those early morning hours. If we determine that we spend the majority of the time asleep and not awake, but we still remain anxious about our sleep, it may be a good idea to practise some CBT to counteract the negative thoughts around sleep and develop some alternative, more positive thoughts like 'Even though it doesn't seem like it to me, I am getting good sleep and it is exactly what I need'.

Adopting a relaxation exercise before bedtime may also help as it prepares our body and mind for sleep. It may be that some worry we have experienced during the day keeps popping up in our light sleep in the morning hours, making us think that we are lying awake thinking about it when in fact it is just snippets of thoughts sifting through our mind when we are asleep.

If you do find out that what you thought was early morning wakefulness was in fact a misperception of your sleep state think of it as good news. It means that while you may be a little frustrated in the early morning hours, thinking you can't sleep, you really are getting the sleep you need and therefore luckily will probably not be suffering all the adverse health outcomes of sleeplessness.

Insomnia due to poor sleep hygiene

This type of insomnia will occur when we do things during our wakeful hours that are inconsistent with good sleep. For example, if we have irregular sleep times, drink coffee late into the night or go for a long run just before we want to sleep. Such activities will wake the brain up and make sleep difficult. Poor sleep hygiene is a relatively common cause of primary insomnia. If you think this may be the cause of your problem it is important that you pay attention to the next chapter.

We have now come to a significant part of the book. We have almost completed our journey through sleep and sleeplessness – its types, its causes and its treatments. You should by now understand the processes of sleep and the differences between primary and secondary insomnia. You should be able to recognise when your sleep difficulties occur – at the beginning, during or at the end of your nightly sleep – and you should no longer find sleep and sleeplessness a mystery. Significantly, you now have at hand a whole raft of potential solutions that will help you resolve your particular sleep difficulties.

There is just one thing to keep in mind. For the benefit of clarity each insomnia type and its causes and treatments have been presented separately and been given its own distinct chapter. Because of this some readers may have developed an idea that this distinct presentation is indicative of what happens in the real world. This is not the case and when we work through our sleep issues we need to keep in mind the numerous stories presented in this book and to remember that many of the people we have learned about had a number of problems that needed to be worked through in a step-by-step manner. As we saw with Rick, while he did have secondary insomnia (due to sleep apnoea) he had also developed a level of primary insomnia (due to bad sleep hygiene) and had trouble both getting to and staying asleep. So for Rick, as it will be for many of us, diagnosing the cause of his insomnia is merely the first step.

The fact that we are able now to make that first step is great news because, as with everything else in life, once we understand and define a problem we are well on our way to solving it and so it is now for our sleep.

Chapter 15

Good sleep practices

THROUGHOUT THIS BOOK I HAVE emphasised the importance of following good sleep practices, or as they are sometimes referred to, good sleep hygiene. Good sleep practices form part of the steps we need to follow if we are to improve our sleep. Many people reading this book will have undoubtedly struggled with sleep for quite some time and would already be aware of these good sleep practices, as they are widely available. I have also written at length about them in my previous book (*The Sleep Diet*). They are, however, an essential topic to discuss in any book dealing with sleep and so I will now discuss them in detail.

Most of us would be able to offer at least one or two sleep tips to help a person who is struggling with sleep. We may not understand why a particular sleep tip will work, but it is almost common knowledge that it will help. There are ten sleep tips that are essential information. If we understand the why and how of these then we are well on our way to having the sleep we want:

1. Maintain a regular bedtime and awakening time.
2. Do not sleep during the day.
3. Avoid alcohol.

4. Avoid caffeinated beverages after noon.
5. Do not smoke before bedtime.
6. Do not exercise within 3 hours of bedtime.
7. Finish eating 2–3 hours before bedtime.
8. Adopt a going-to-bed routine.
9. Do not use the bed or bedroom for anything other than sleep and sexual activity.
10. Keep the bedroom cool, dark, quiet and comfortable.

Following these practices will help us sleep better because they prevent us from disrupting the circadian rhythms that are so critical to our sleep and they also enhance the harmonisation of these rhythms so that we get consolidated sleep. Over the course of this chapter we will discuss each of these practices individually so that by the end we will hopefully understand not just the practice itself but the 'why' of the practice – and in that way we increase the likelihood that we will stick to each practice.

Maintain a regular bedtime and awakening time

Regular going-to-bed and waking-up times strengthen our circadian cycles and make going to sleep at night much easier. An erratic bedtime schedule will impact significantly on the quality and quantity of sleep and will frequently result in insufficient sleep, causing all the consequences we have learned about.

Mary's story

Mary, an executive of an international mining company, was experiencing difficulty getting to sleep. No matter how tired she was she just could not get to sleep quickly. Whether she went to bed early or late, she would often toss and turn for up to an hour, or longer, before she fell asleep. Once asleep she slept well but because she had to get up early the next day, she frequently got much less sleep than she wanted (and needed).

Mary's job required her frequently to be up late at night for conference calls and on occasion she needed to travel overseas for short periods of time. Her working schedule disrupted her sleep so much that when asked what her normal bedtime was Mary was at a loss. When pressed, she thought her bedtime was any time between 9 pm and 1 am, and even though most days she needed to be up by 7 am she would often sleep in due to her tiredness, and she would especially take the opportunity to sleep in on weekends. Mary was tired and irritable and thought that if she could get to sleep when she went to bed then everything would be fine and she would be able to get the amount of sleep she desired.

Mary did not understand the process of her daily biological rhythms. On the nights she stayed up late for work she normally worked in her study, which was brightly lit. She would also be working on her computer, which again was brightly lit. The amount of light Mary's eyes were detecting from both her computer and the overhead light meant that her brain was unable to discern the fading daylight and therefore did not register the fact that it was time to start secreting melatonin – our very important sleep hormone.

This meant that not only was her melatonin cycle pushed back – such that she did not start to secrete melatonin until much later (when she dimmed the lights) – but it also had the flow-on effect of delaying other biological rhythms (phase delay). As a consequence, the following night, despite Mary not working late and wanting to go to bed a little earlier, both her daily temperature cycle and her daily alerting cycle were delayed, which meant they were out of sync with her melatonin secretion, causing Mary to toss and turn for an hour or so before her temperature and alertness began to decrease – allowing for sleep.

If Mary only had the odd irregular bedtime she would have had just the odd night of disturbed sleep and she could have managed this. But it was a common occurrence and it meant that her body's cycles were not in harmony. Since her going-to-bed time and her getting-up time were forever changing Mary suffered from an extremely poor sleeping pattern.

Mary loved her job and was not about to change it so she needed advice as to how to improve her sleep. Many of us are in Mary's position, but this does not mean we are doomed to poor sleep. By recognising the problem – disrupted circadian cycles – we can start to do something constructive.

Firstly, Mary was advised to negotiate a bedtime that was within reasonable limits – no later than 11 pm – and establish a regular getting-up time, somewhere between 7–7.30 am. Secondly, she was advised to work under dim lights and, even if she had to stay up late for a conference call, she needed to switch off her computer an hour before the call. By doing this she was allowing her brain to detect fading light and thus start secretion of melatonin so that by the end of her conference call her melatonin would have reached a sufficient level to encourage sleep. Thirdly, she was encouraged to have a hot shower (but not so hot that she was overheated) after the call – and only then go to bed. In this way Mary was creating a falling body temperature – something which further enhanced feelings of sleepiness.

Mary's sleep did improve – and even on the nights that it did not (due to her extremely erratic sleep times) she understood the reason why she was unable to sleep, thereby decreasing the exasperation she had felt in the past about her inability to fall asleep. This latter point is important. When we don't sleep well we often feel frustrated, and if our poor sleep continues over a number of nights many of us will start to stress. As we have discussed previously, this just increases the likelihood of poor sleep. By understanding the processes of sleep we can begin to understand what lies at the heart of the poor sleep and how we can begin to change it.

Do not sleep during the day

For the purposes of this sleep practice it is necessary to distinguish between a sleep and a nap. A nap is in effect a short sleep period of about 20 minutes. A sleep, on the other hand, is longer than this and often involves a full sleep cycle (lasting up to 90 minutes). For many of us napping through the day causes no problem; indeed it may be particularly helpful when we have not been able to get sufficient sleep in the previous few nights because of, for example, a sick child. As we have seen previously, a nap taken during our afternoon lull period can be effective in waking us up and allowing us to be alert until it is time to go to bed that night.

For others, a nap can turn into a sleep and this can cause significant problems with the night-time sleep. For Mac, this certainly was a problem.

Mac's story

Mac was a freelance journalist and worked from home. This had worked well until the birth of his son 2 years ago. Soon after the birth, Mac's partner resumed work. As she worked a 9–5 job in an office it was decided that Mac could look after the baby when the baby awoke during the night as Mac would have more of an opportunity to catch up on sleep during the day. Since Mac also had his freelance work to do, it often meant that he would have to work late into the night (once the baby was asleep) and he frequently got only 5–6 hours' sleep during the night. This left him incredibly tired during the day and he would often have a sleep (up to 2 hours) in the afternoon, when his wife got home from work, to tide him over. While this strategy worked for a while, and was especially useful when his son was younger, it was not working as well now that the child was sleeping consistently throughout the night and Mac could have got 8 hours during the night-time if he was able to. Unfortunately though, Mac had got into the habit of an afternoon sleep.

Despite the fact that he had reduced his daytime sleep to around 40–50 minutes, he was finding it increasingly difficult to get to sleep at night and, as a result, was only averaging about 6 hours. Mac realised that his afternoon sleep was probably not helping but, because he was so tired, it was almost impossible not to fall asleep in the afternoon.

By understanding the process of sleep – the balancing of our sleep drive against our circadian rhythms – we can understand why Mac was finding initiating sleep at night so difficult. After he slept in the afternoon Mac felt much more awake. This was because, by sleeping, he decreased the amount of sleep chemicals in his brain and thereby decreased his sleep drive. So, while he felt brighter and more awake, which was good, he also effectively decreased his sleep drive so that when it got to 11 pm – a time when he should have gone to sleep – he was unable to. It was taking Mac until much later to get to sleep, often around 1 am.

By looking at the diagram below you can see how Mac's afternoon sleep (black dotted line) caused maximal sleep drive to occur later – at which time Mac would drop off to sleep.

The problem was that Mac's getting-up time didn't change by much so he had not managed to normalise his sleep drive by the time he needed to get up. As a consequence he ended up needing the afternoon sleep the next day.

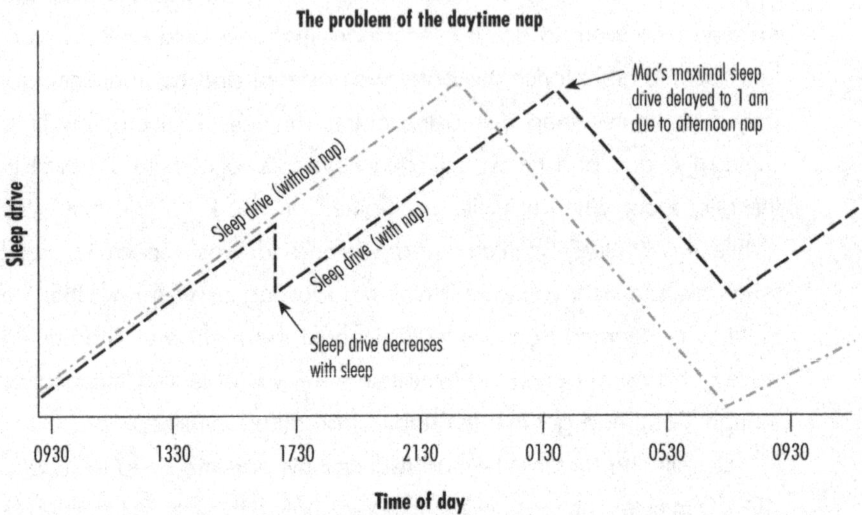

For Mac, this cycle was difficult to break as he found it extremely difficult not to fall asleep during the latter part of the afternoon. Once he began to understand just how finely modulated sleep really is, and how it is an interaction of a number of rhythms, Mac could see the relevance of making a few changes and sticking with them.

Mac needed to improve two aspects of his sleep. Firstly, he needed to exchange his afternoon sleep for an afternoon nap. Secondly, he needed to change how he went about his work in the evening so that he enhanced the harmony of his biological rhythms and would feel tired at the time that he needed to go to bed (around 11 pm).

To successfully change from a sleep to a nap in the afternoon Mac worked out (by using the alerting cycle exercise in Chapter 3) what time he normally felt the sleepiest in the afternoon. At that time he would lie down on the sofa and have an alarm set to go off 20 minutes later. Once the alarm went off he would get up and undertake some exercise, outdoors if possible. This could be as simple as taking the baby for a walk around the block. Even if Mac did not fall asleep within 20 minutes he still got up once the alarm sounded and did something active. By doing this Mac was able to manage his extreme afternoon tiredness without excessively decreasing his sleep drive.

In order to change his nightly routine, Mac made sure that the lights in the room were dimmed an hour before his scheduled bedtime, and that his computer and tablet were switched off so that he could not be distracted by work.

Within a week, by implementing these strategies, Mac was able to fall asleep within 10–15 minutes of going to bed and was able to maintain his sleep until his normal wake-up time. As his night-time sleep gradually improved, Mac's need for the afternoon nap decreased and before too long he had dispensed with it altogether, although he still exercised around his afternoon lull.

While Mac was only 34 years old, his problem – the need to sleep during the day – is often seen in older people.

Many of us, as we get older, have less to do with our day and our daytime busyness decreases. This can be especially true for retired people who, instead of being fully occupied at work during their afternoon dip in alertness, are now free to do what they desire. If they are in a passive situation in the mid-afternoon when their alertness level is low, they may nod off and have an afternoon sleep. If they are not careful they will then find themselves in the same situation as Mac – not being able to sleep that night.

So if you are unemployed or retired and you find it difficult to fall asleep at night, don't immediately jump to the conclusion that it is a result of anxiety or the ageing process – it may merely be the poor sleep practice that you have inadvertently started to adopt.

Avoid alcohol

If you are experiencing any difficulty sleeping, alcohol is definitely not recommended. We have already dealt with this in great detail in Chapter 13 so I will not discuss it further here. If you are one of the 10% of people whose sleep problem is caused by alcohol, please take special note of Chapter 13.

Avoid caffeinated beverages after noon

Caffeine is a potent stimulant and, as we discovered in Chapter 3, it works by blocking the effect of the sleepy chemical, adenosine. The longer we are awake the higher the level of brain adenosine, and the sleepier we become.

Caffeine prevents the brain from recognising the level of adenosine thereby masking our level of tiredness. Caffeine is probably the most widely available stimulant, used to better our mood, increase our alertness and to improve our thinking processes.

While caffeine use can be a distinct advantage when we are tired and need to be alert and thinking well, it obviously makes sleeping difficult. It is therefore important to understand some of the chemical properties of caffeine to ensure that it always works to our advantage rather than working against us.

A cup of coffee takes about 30 minutes to have an effect – and the maximum effect is experienced about an hour after drinking it at which point the level of caffeine peaks in our blood. After this time there is a decline in the level of caffeine but it takes at least 3 hours (and sometimes up to 7 hours) to halve caffeine blood levels. In other words, our one cup of coffee (which typically contains about 100 mg of caffeine) is still having an effect up to 5 hours later when there is still about 50 mg of caffeine in our blood.

This means that if we have a cup of coffee at 6 pm, 5 hours later at 11 pm we will still have 50 mg of caffeine in our blood – and this remaining amount may well and truly affect our ability to initiate sleep.

How much caffeine remains in our system and for how long depends upon our metabolic rate. Our metabolic rate decreases with age so that in our forties and fifties coffee in the late afternoon can very much affect our ability to sleep, whereas it may have had minimal impact on us when we were younger. Therefore, the older we get the more likely it is that caffeine becomes a contributor to our sleeplessness. Most of us fall into the trap of thinking that because caffeine has not been problematic in the past, it is not now the cause for our sleeplessness despite the fact that we may be 20 years older and our metabolic rate significantly slower. This means that we need to start considering whether caffeine – and all types of caffeine consumption, including tea, coffee, energy drinks, soft drinks and chocolate – is, in part, responsible for our sleepless nights.

If we are still under the effects of caffeine when we go to bed we will have trouble initiating sleep and trouble maintaining our deep sleep. To overcome this, caffeine, in any form, should only be had in the morning hours, and any afternoon caffeine needs to be restricted. If you are currently consuming a lot of caffeine reducing your intake may need to be done gradually as some withdrawal effects such as headache, increased tiredness and worsened mood may be experienced. These symptoms may be evident within the first day of caffeine reduction but are only transitory.

Do not smoke before bedtime

For many of those who smoke, a relaxing cigarette before bedtime is a common habit. Nicotine makes smokers feel good. It stimulates the reward pathways in the brain, causing the smoker to feel relaxed and happy. It also stimulates production of endorphins, often referred to as the 'euphoria hormones'. As a result a 'calming' cigarette before bedtime is often considered to induce relaxation and therefore sleep.

This is incorrect. While nicotine does promote the feel-good pathways in the brain, it is a stimulant and initially causes a rapid release of adrenaline and an increase in heart rate, blood pressure, metabolic and breathing rates – which is the complete opposite to preparing the body for sleep. Nicotine also causes the brain to produce a particular chemical, acetylcholine, which increases brain activity. As opposed to adenosine, which is our sleepy chemical, acetylcholine is important in maintaining our wakefulness, and this is what many smokers rely upon to re-energise themselves throughout the day.

It is not surprising therefore that numerous studies have shown that smokers have a higher prevalence of sleep disturbances than non-smokers. Various studies have shown that smokers experience insomnia-like symptoms, including difficulty getting to sleep, difficulty waking up, non-restorative sleep, difficulty staying asleep, excessive daytime sleepiness, and decreased total sleep time. If you are trying to optimise your sleep it is highly recommended to quit smoking (of course there are also numerous other reasons why this is a good idea). Quitting smoking will frequently cause withdrawal symptoms such as irritability, anxiety, depression and cravings for nicotine – all of which may exacerbate any sleep problems in the short term. Be reassured, however, that by understanding the processes of sleep and optimising the functioning of your circadian cycle you will be able to minimise these withdrawal effects, and they will subside over 2–4 weeks.

For those of you who have decided to stick with smoking, it is important to minimise its effect on your sleep. Nicotine has a rapid effect on our body. While it takes caffeine up to half an hour for its effects to be felt, the effects of nicotine are felt within 10–15 seconds of the first inhalation. Unlike caffeine, its half-life is relatively short – about 60 minutes – which means that within 5 hours there is almost no nicotine in the body. Indeed, it is the withdrawal of nicotine from the system while the smoker sleeps that is thought to cause the myriad of sleep disturbances.

If we realise that the effect of nicotine is rapid and that nicotine will increase our alertness and re-energise us, the worst thing we could do is have a cigarette just before bed. This will completely sabotage all of our best efforts for good sleep. So, even if you have decided not to quit smoking, in order to maximise your chances of having good consolidated sleep, then at the very least you should not smoke within 2 hours of bedtime.

Do not exercise within 3 hours of bedtime

In the next chapter we will talk about the benefits of exercise on our sleep – however for now we are just going to look at the potential exercise has to disrupt sleep. If exercise is not to cause problems for your sleep it has to be done at the right intensity and at the right time.

While there is still a lot of research and discussion about what time of day or what level of intensity promotes the best sleep, what is clear is that if we exercise after about 6 pm at night it is highly likely that it will have a negative impact on our ability to get to sleep. This is because by exercising we are not only increasing our core body temperature (and thereby upsetting our circadian rhythm of temperature) but we are also increasing our heart rate, blood pressure and metabolic rate – all of which increase our level of alertness and thereby upset our circadian rhythm of alertness. We are also affecting another of our biological rhythms which is important in our sleep-wake cycle – that of cortisol.

We have already spoken about our stress response in chapters 5 and 6 and the fact that when we are stressed we produce cortisol, along with adrenaline and noradrenaline.

Cortisol is also important in managing our transition from sleep to wakefulness and its secretion profile is opposite to that of melatonin. Cortisol starts to rise in the dawn hours (as melatonin begins to decrease) and is highest in the early morning (6–8 am) and lowest at around midnight (when melatonin is at a maximum). If melatonin is considered to be our sleepy hormone, cortisol could be thought of as our wakeful hormone. The circadian profile of cortisol secretion is important in allowing us to be awake in the morning hours and not awake in the dark hours. What has been found though is that cortisol levels will increase in response to exercise. So if we exercise in the night hours, when our cortisol is meant to be decreasing (in order to allow melatonin to do its job), it may be difficult to get to sleep that night.

Timing of exercise is also something to keep in mind if you suffer from Delayed Sleep Phase Syndrome (DSPS). While it is not understood why, exercising in the late afternoon advances our body clock by up to 30 minutes. This results in a phase advance that can be used advantageously for people like Charlotte who have DSPS or even the owls amongst us who just want to get to sleep a little earlier. By exercising in the late afternoon, but no later than 6 pm, you will advance your body clock a little and often find that you are able to get to sleep about 30 minutes earlier than usual.

While exercising at the right time is a critical factor in maximising the beneficial sleep effects so too is the level of exercise intensity. If, after learning about all the wonderful positive aspects of exercise on our sleep, we decide to go out and do some exercise we must make sure we do not overdo it. Many of us may not have exercised for months or maybe even years. Despite this, we might make the mistake of doing an intense workout on our first day back in the gym. Not surprisingly many of us will discover muscles we never even knew existed and, rather than enhancing our sleep, our sleep will be disturbed due to the aches and pains we are experiencing. Far better that we slowly introduce exercise into our daily routine as we have seen others do throughout this book. For example, it may be that getting off the bus a stop or two earlier is a good way to start, or a 20-minute walk three or four times a week for the first few weeks, gradually increasing our pace. Once we have acquired a level of fitness we can introduce more strenuous exercise.

Finish eating 2–3 hours before bedtime

Eating or drinking too close to bedtime may have a detrimental effect on our ability to get to sleep and to maintain our sleep.

Alex's story

Alex and his wife Michelle decided to make a tree-change. They sold their house in the city and invested in a small property in the country. While they were very happy with their decision and were mostly enjoying their new lifestyle, there were a few drawbacks, the most notable being the time it took Alex to get to and from work. While he planned on relocating his work eventually, he needed to keep his city job in the short term.

This meant that during the week he had to go to the city, which was a 2.5-hour commute each way. Most days Alex left home at about 5.45 am (having woken up at 5 am) and didn't arrive back home until at least 7.30 pm. Dinner was invariably around 8.30 pm after which Alex would relax for about 30 minutes before dropping into bed exhausted. Sadly, Alex was finding it increasingly difficult to get to sleep. He would toss and turn for at least an hour before eventually going into a fitful sleep.

Needless to say Alex's poor sleep was affecting his ability to enjoy his new country life. Most mornings he awoke unrefreshed and he was finding that he was spending most of his weekend just catching up on sleep. Alex had rarely experienced any difficulties with his sleep in the past. He thought that perhaps his new difficulties with sleeping were associated with the stress accompanying his lifestyle change and he was looking for ways to help him better manage this stress.

While Alex's poor sleep may have had something to do with the new changes in his life, a large part of his sleeping problems was directly attributable to his eating pattern. Having a large meal (his main meal of the day) just an hour before he went to bed meant that Alex was continually being disturbed by the process of digesting his food.

Many people give little consideration to the timing of their evening meal – and yet it can have a significant negative impact on our ability to have good sleep. After we eat, our digestive system works to break down the food in order for us to use it for energy or store it as fat. This digestive process increases our metabolic rate which in turn increases our body temperature. With an increase in temperature we will find it difficult to sleep (remember we like to fall asleep on a decreasing temperature). So, eating a large meal within about 2–3 hours of bedtime can cause difficulties in initiating sleep.

The problems with eating and sleep do not involve just the problem of getting to sleep. As with many of our biological systems our gastrointestinal system also has a 24-hour cycle, which slows down during sleep. As a consequence of this slow-down it is unable to digest the food as quickly as it would if we were awake and active. This means that a meal that would ordinarily take 2–3 hours to be emptied from the stomach will take considerably longer. In the process, not only will we experience a level of discomfort due to the increased gastric volume but we will also experience substantial difficulties in getting into our deep sleep.

While the process of digestion itself will interfere with our attempts to have good sleep we may also find that we will suffer more from heartburn (or reflux). This will lead to further difficulty with falling asleep and cause ongoing discomfort throughout the night.

Anyone who suffers from reflux knows just how unpleasant it is. When we eat, food passes from the mouth into the oesophagus and then into the stomach where it is mixed with acid to aid digestion. Normally, food only goes one way and is prevented from going back into the oesophagus by means of a valve at the entrance to the stomach. For some people, this valve does not work effectively and some stomach contents may be regurgitated into the oesophagus. At this stage the food contents are acidic and will cause considerable burning in the oesophagus – which is why reflux is often referred to as heartburn. While many of us suffer from heartburn even when awake and upright, any tendency to reflux will be greatly exacerbated when lying down. Even those of us who do not ordinarily suffer from reflux may find we do so if we lie down after a large meal – as the forces of gravity may well overcome the capability of the valve.

When Alex became aware of how he was sabotaging his sleep through his eating pattern he realised that he had to make a concerted effort to change.

Alex began having his main meal of the day at lunchtime. On his journey home he would have a light meal (equivalent to what he used to have for lunch) and when he arrived home in the evening he would have a light snack around 8 pm. By adopting these small changes, Alex was able to go to bed at 9.30 pm, fall asleep generally within 15 minutes and sleep solidly until 5 am the next day. He felt life was worth living again and that their move to the country was indeed the right one.

It is also worthwhile to note how much liquid we consume before bedtime. Even though our kidney function slows down over night and we do not produce as much urine, if we drink too much too late in the evening we will need to get up during the night to urinate and this will interrupt our sleep. As we age the tendency to pass urine during the night (referred to as nocturia) increases. If you find that drinking a cup of herbal tea before bedtime causes you to get up during the night it would be a good idea to forgo the cup of tea, even if previously it had been part of your go-to-bed routine.

Adopt a going-to-bed routine

One of the most vital ingredients to a good night's sleep is the establishment of a going-to-bed routine. If this is done well it will ensure that all the circadian rhythms are in synchrony and that when we go to bed we will be able to fall asleep easily.

A going-to-bed routine could involve any or all of the following:

1. At least an hour before going to bed, dim the lights. Studies have shown that we are most sensitive to light during the dark

hours and lights at night will delay our circadian rhythm and therefore the onset of melatonin secretion, creating difficulty initiating sleep.

2. Switch off any computers – this will have a twofold effect. Firstly, by having the computer on, our eyes are focused on a strong light which has the effect of delaying melatonin secretion. Secondly, generally, if we are at the computer, we are undertaking some thinking task. If we are thinking hard we are increasing our level of alertness at a time when we want to have minimal alertness – remember our circadian rhythm of alertness needs to be on the decline to allow us to easily go to sleep.
3. Have a hot shower half an hour before bed. This has the effect of passively increasing the body's temperature, so that after showering the body will start to cool down, mimicking the decline of temperature seen ordinarily in our daily temperature cycle. Not only will this enhance the effect of sleepiness experienced due to a declining temperature, but it should also have the added benefit of relieving some of the muscle tension that may have built up during the day.
4. Do a relaxation exercise. For some of us, dimming the lights, switching off the computer or having a hot shower is not sufficient to switch off our brain. In this case it is often beneficial to do some form of relaxation practice – this could involve any one of the practices that were discussed in Chapter 6.
5. Start a 'worry diary'. We have spoken about this previously and it is an effective way of dealing with the issues that arise during the day. In times of particular stress, when there seem to be so many problems to solve, we will often go to bed and mull over issues even when the thing we most want to do is sleep. One of the reasons this happens is that during busy times the only time we have an opportunity to do big-picture problem solving is in the quiet of the bedroom – when we really need to be sleeping.

It is helpful when we first arrive home, or at some other time during the evening (but at least an hour and a half before bedtime), to write down all the problems of the day – at least the ones concerning us most. We may even choose to note possible solutions alongside each of these. We should give ourselves no more than half an hour to do this as it is at the end of a long day and our thinking processes may not be working at their best. Far better to write down any problems and work on them after a good night's sleep. As many of us know by experience, problems often seem far more worrisome and insolvable late at night than they do after a good sleep.

The need for a going-to-bed routine should not be minimised. It will certainly maximise the opportunity for getting to sleep and staying asleep even when we are under considerable stress.

Do not use the bed or bedroom for anything other than sleep and sexual activity

The bedroom is not the place for televisions, computers or work material of any kind. It is important that there is nothing in the bedroom to cause an increase in our alertness or anxiety (this may well be something as seemingly benign as the bedroom clock). Not only does this ensure that we do not disturb our biological movement towards sleep but it also ensures that we entrain a conditioning response to the association between bed and sleep.

Most of us have heard, at some time or other, the story of Pavlov and his dogs. Pavlov was a Russian scientist in the late 19th century. Amongst his many discoveries was the fact that dogs developed a 'conditioned' response to the sound of a bell. Normally when dogs sense food they will start to produce saliva. This is important as it aids in the digestion of the food. What Pavlov found though was that if he struck a bell whenever the dogs were fed, eventually the dogs would begin to salivate just at the sound of the bell, even in the absence of food. This kind of learned response is called a conditioned reflex, and the process of learning to connect a particular stimulus to a reflex is called conditioning.

Humans as well as dogs are susceptible to conditioning – and many of us have experienced it quite simply when we have eaten something and have been coincidentally sick afterwards. Even though the food was not necessarily responsible for the illness suffered we will be sufficiently conditioned not to want to eat that particular food again.

Our susceptibility to conditioning can work against us if we are unaware of the effect it can have on our ability to go to sleep. If every night we go to bed only to watch television for an hour or so, or to do some work, we are inadvertently conditioning ourselves to stay awake for up to an hour every time we go to bed. As a result, on the nights we go to bed and want to go to sleep immediately we will find it very difficult.

For many of us TV in the bedroom has become a fact of life – much to our unsuspecting detriment. We need to get rid of the TV, computer, study books and any other work-related paraphernalia from our bedroom.

There is some good news though. It would seem that while most activities conducted in the bedroom (like watching TV and playing on the computer) will result in negative conditioning for our sleep, sexual activity in the bedroom does not cause the same issues. In fact, research shows us that, contrary to the regular advice about not exercising within 3 hours of bedtime, sexual activity actually enhances our propensity to sleep.

So why is that? Obviously, sex usually increases the heart rate and blood pressure and certainly body temperature starts to rise – all those things that we have learned will work against us when we try to go to sleep. Many of us, however, feel very sleepy after sex and there are a number of reasons why this is so.

Firstly, in order to orgasm, we need to be able to let go of fear and anxiety. This release of stress relaxes us, and for many will be sufficient to promote sleep. Additionally though when we orgasm there is a release of a lot of brain chemicals, including a number that are directly associated with sleep. Primary amongst these is prolactin, which is naturally released during sleep and enhances sleep, and oxytocin, which actively decreases our stress levels, again increasing the likelihood of sleep.

So it would seem that sex is not just any exercise, but a very special one, releasing all sorts of wonderful chemicals that relax us and make us feel good. And, unlike other exercise, it is a good thing to do just prior to going to sleep.

Keep the bedroom cool, dark, quiet and comfortable

The fact that the bedroom environment is the last of the sleep practices I am going to discuss does not imply that it has a low priority. A healthy sleep environment is critical in maintaining sleep and there are a number of 'must-haves' for your bedroom:

1. The bedroom must be dark. If the room is light, we will not produce enough melatonin to keep us asleep. Some of us may be able to sleep in a not-so-dark room but for others it will be very difficult. It is sometimes surprising to see just how susceptible some people are to the alerting effects of light – indeed research has shown that even very dim light (a candle or a digital clock) can cause problems for some people. To create a dark environment either blackout blinds or eye masks work well.
2. The bedroom must be quiet. Sleep is difficult to maintain in a noisy environment. This makes sense in an evolutionary way, as it would have been dangerous for cavemen to continue sleeping when there were marauding tribes outside the cave. At that time, the awakening response to noise was a protective phenomenon. In modern society we no longer live in caves and generally sleep in fairly secure environments – nevertheless, we still have a strong arousal response to noise.

   Luckily for us, our ability to be conditioned can work in our favour and we frequently become conditioned not to wake up to a known noise such as snoring. We learn to habituate to the snoring because over time we find that the snoring does not place us in danger and therefore it is safe not to wake up in response to it. However, the fact that we learn not to wake in response to this or any other noise does not mean that the noise has no effect on our sleep. Indeed, while we may sleep through the noise, studies examining the effects of noise on sleep have shown that it will increase our arousal level, fragment sleep and lead to reduction in the time spent in deep sleep and REM sleep, typically increasing the time we spend in light sleep. This means that we not only wake up unrefreshed the next day, but we will also experience the hormonal, cognitive and behavioural deficits that accompany fragmented sleep.

In order to minimise the effect of noise on our sleep it may be advisable to wear earplugs or to have some form of white noise machine. White noise contains all (or most) noise frequencies and is able to mask other sounds. Surprisingly a standard fan produces a good approximation of white noise and is an easy thing to have in the bedroom.

It is important to evaluate the effect of environmental noise on your sleep. If your partner snores or you live in a noisy traffic area, be particularly aware of the effect this may be having on you and your ability to sleep well. A good pair of earplugs or a fan can make a remarkable difference.

3. The bedroom needs to be at an appropriate temperature. The temperature of our bedroom has a big influence on our ability to maintain sleep. As we have learned, we have a tendency to arouse on an increasing temperature and so if the room is too hot then we will have trouble maintaining sleep and our sleep will become fragmented. On the other hand, if the room is too cold we won't be able to sustain our REM sleep because in this stage of sleep we can't shiver (remember that in REM sleep we are paralysed except for our breathing muscles), and if we can't shiver we can't maintain our core temperature. Indeed, most of us would have at some stage experienced this inability to maintain our body temperature in REM sleep when we have woken up in the early hours of the morning needing to put on an extra blanket.

Sometimes, especially if we share our bedroom with someone else, it is difficult to decide on the correct temperature for our best sleep. Research tells us that the ideal temperature for sleeping is around 18°C, but because we are all individuals it is worthwhile experimenting to find out exactly what temperature suits us and our partner. Often a fan, which may also be used as a white-noise generator, is effective in cooling down a room sufficiently to make sleeping more comfortable.

4. Our mattress must be comfortable and supportive. There is almost no point in discussing good sleep practices if your bed is uncomfortable. So many of us take our bed for granted and end up using it for far too many years – often past its use-by date. A non-supportive bed can result in considerable discomfort throughout the night and chronic back pain throughout the day. Most of us use our bed for at least 7–9 hours in every 24 hours, so our need for a good bed is absolute. Most mattresses have a life expectancy of 9 or 10 years. If we have been using one for longer than this, it needs to be changed. Even if we have not had it for this length of time but it is uncomfortable and causing difficulty with sleeping, we need to upgrade to the most comfortable one we can afford as soon as possible. Comfortable pillows are also a necessity and it is worthwhile investing in the best ones we can afford. Many people suffer from neck pain that affects both their sleep and wakeful hours and which is, unknown to them, a direct consequence of poor pillow support.
5. The bedroom should be harmonious to our needs. Once we have a comfortable bed and pillow, and the bedroom is dark, quiet and cool, we are almost ready to use it for sleep. I say 'almost' because there is one last thing we may need to do. For some of us our bedroom needs to be reflective of our personality and harmonious to our needs. Many of us need to be able to enter the bedroom and feel an immediate sense of peace and relaxation. For these people investing energy into the right design and interior decoration of the bedroom may be important.

   On the other hand, others amongst us can have the messiest bedrooms and still sleep soundly. So, if a messy room does not cause us any anxious moments and we find that it is, regardless of the mess or the colour, a room that we sleep well in, then we can discard this last bit of advice and just go ahead and enjoy our newfound sleep.

This brings me to my last point about the need for good sleep habits. Sleep is meant to be something to be enjoyed, to look forward to at the end of a long day. It is meant to make us feel refreshed and energised to meet the new day. It is a process which, if we allow it, will come naturally. Many of us have, over the years, gradually degraded our opportunity for good sleep without realising that this was what we were doing. If we are now serious about reclaiming our sleep then implementing these sleep practices is critical. Integrating all ten of these practices into the routine of our life may take time but once we manage to do this we will benefit greatly from our ability to get deep, restful sleep.

Chapter 16

Sleep and a healthy lifestyle

OVER THE LAST 30 YEARS we have begun to unquestioningly accept that without good food and good exercise we will not have good health. It is now also recognised by many of us that our health is critically affected by how we sleep. The idea that there are three pillars of health is also gaining more and more credence in the medical world. It is still early days though and we are still discovering some of the important interactions between sleeping, eating and exercising. In this chapter we are going to look at some of these interactions and find out what, if any, changes we need to make to our approach to eating and exercising to maximise our potential for good, restful sleep.

Exercise

There is now more than enough scientific evidence confirming how beneficial exercise is for our overall good health. One of the marvellous things about exercise is that it has been shown to increase the amount of growth hormone we produce. Growth hormone has been likened to the 'fountain of youth' and is integral to how well we are able to maintain and repair our body. Typically, growth hormone is secreted in our sleep and we have a spike in its secretion in the first half of our sleep, when we have most of our deep sleep.

As we grow older the amount of growth hormone in our body decreases and our ability to maintain and repair our body declines. The good news is that exercise produces an increase in growth hormone secretion during sleep and older people who exercise have higher levels of growth hormone. This valuable effect of exercise on our health has been known for some time now but what has been more recently discovered is that exercising directly affects our ability to sleep soundly. In numerous large surveys it has been found that exercise is the most nominated factor for improving sleep quality, and people who exercise regularly experience less daytime tiredness. The more exercise someone performs, the better the quality of sleep. Studies have also confirmed that there is a lower prevalence of self-reported sleep problems and daytime sleepiness in physically active people compared to more sedentary people. In fact, it has been shown that exercise confers many beneficial effects on our sleep, including decreasing the time it takes for us to get to sleep and increasing both our total sleep time and the amount of time we spend in deep sleep.

Importantly, the same positive effects of exercise are observed with either light, moderate or intense exercise. Clearly, exercise is excellent for promoting sleep and is an important component to consider if we are having difficulties sleeping.

Nutrition

It is not just exercise that improves our sleep but also what we put into our bodies. Our food provides all the proteins, vitamins and minerals necessary to produce the hormones that promote the sleep pathways in our brain, which allow us to get to sleep and to stay asleep. While some foods can actively enhance our sleep, other foods can actively steal it (as we have already seen with caffeine), and so when we are seeking to optimise our sleep it is important to know which foods do what. Later in the chapter we will look at some of the more common food items that can rob us of sleep, but right now, we are going to find out what we can eat in order to give us the best sleep possible.

Foods that enhance sleep

To understand how what we eat can help us sleep, we need to understand the chemistry of sleep. If we recall that melatonin is our sleepy hormone, and its production is essential to our sleep, it makes sense that those foods that contribute to the making of melatonin will enhance our sleep. The diagram below shows how melatonin is produced by the body. This diagram makes it clear that our body needs particular proteins, vitamins and minerals. How we get these and which particular foods provide these ingredients in abundance is important for the optimisation of our sleep.

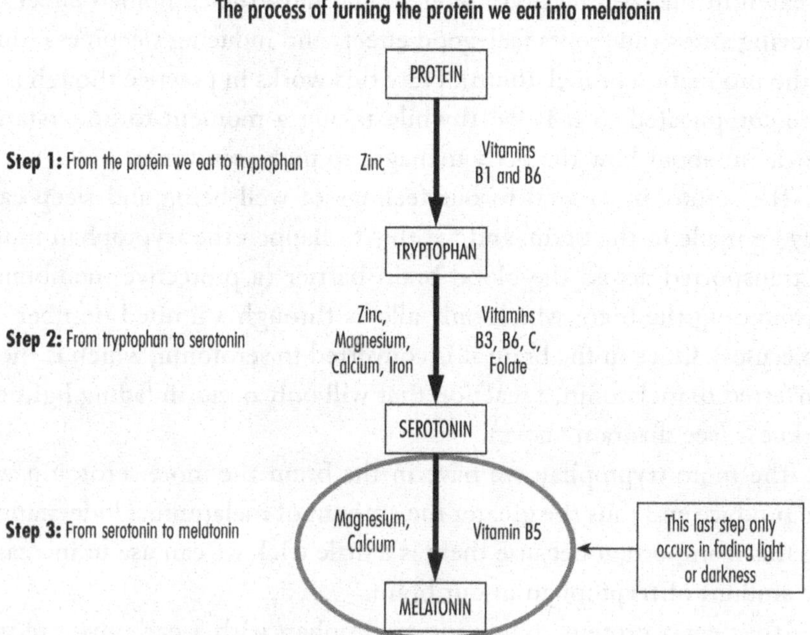

Protein and Tryptophan

When we eat protein it is broken down into compounds called amino acids. There are 22 known amino acids and they form the building blocks for our body's protein as well as being essential for a vast array of bodily processes, including those necessary for sleeping and wakefulness. Tryptophan is one of these amino acids and is found in most of the proteins we eat but the amount present depends on the type of protein.

It comes in two forms, D- and L-, but the L form is more common and is the one found in the proteins in the body.

Tryptophan is essential to our sleep because, as we can see from the above diagram, it is the primary building block for serotonin (our feel-good hormone) and melatonin. Tryptophan is thought of by many as a natural hypnotic substance and it has been shown that increasing tryptophan increases the amounts of both serotonin and melatonin, decreasing the time it takes us to get to sleep (sleep latency) and increasing deep sleep – all great news for those of us trying to optimise our sleep.

As a consequence of its positive effect on mood and sleep, it is often recommended that protein containing high levels of tryptophan be eaten in the evening hours as it should have the combined effect of relieving stress (due to its feel-good effect) and inducing sleepiness (due to the production of melatonin). How this works in practice though is a little complicated so it is worthwhile taking a moment to understand a little bit about how the body manages to make serotonin.

The serotonin so vital to our feelings of well-being and sleep can only be made in the brain, and for this to happen the tryptophan must be transported across the blood brain barrier (a protective membrane surrounding the brain which only allows through a limited number of molecules). Once in the brain it is converted to serotonin, which is then converted to melatonin, a reaction that will only occur in fading light or darkness (see diagram above).

The more tryptophan we have in the brain the more serotonin we can produce and thus the greater the amount of melatonin. Understanding this is important because there is a little trick we can use to increase the amount of tryptophan in our brain.

If we eat a protein containing tryptophan with a carbohydrate we will increase the amount of tryptophan that can get into our brain. This is the secret to warm milk – the old wives' remedy for insomnia. Milk has a good amount of tryptophan, but it also contains a carbohydrate – the sugar lactose – which enhances the transport of tryptophan into our brain. This in turn promotes the manufacture of serotonin and melatonin, leaving us feeling relaxed and sleepy.

Other good sources of dietary tryptophan are fish, poultry, eggs, dairy products, oatmeal, bananas, nuts and seeds. We can also supplement our diet with L-tryptophan (although I always think fresh is best) and one of the highest sources of supplementary L-tryptophan is alpha-lactalbumin available in health food shops. Studies have shown that taking this supplement in the evening improves sleep and increases early morning alertness the following day, presumably due to the improved sleep.

Vitamins and minerals

To appreciate the relevance of vitamins and minerals in helping us sleep it is important to understand the role they play in making melatonin. As we have just seen, tryptophan is the basic building block for melatonin. But, as the diagram above shows, before melatonin can be made, the protein that we eat must first be broken down into its component parts, including tryptophan, which then must be turned into serotonin and then serotonin converted into melatonin. For each of these steps to occur there needs to be numerous 'helpers' along the way (in the form of vitamins and minerals) and they must be present in the right amounts. If we are deficient in any of these nutrients it will limit the amount of tryptophan that can be produced and therefore the amount of serotonin and melatonin that is made will also be decreased, which has obvious ramifications for our mood and sleep quality. Below we will look at which vitamins are needed for each step, and which foods contain those vitamins.

Step 1: From protein to tryptophan

The first step in making melatonin is the breakdown of the protein we eat into amino acids and specifically into tryptophan. For this to happen our body requires the mineral zinc, and the vitamins B1 and B6.

Zinc: Zinc is essential for the manufacture of melatonin, but it also has an antidepressant activity (due to its role in the manufacture of serotonin) and has been shown to significantly improve sleep quality and mood in older people. While it's uncommon for anyone to be seriously deficient in zinc, lower than normal zinc levels may be seen in the elderly, those with high caffeine or alcohol consumption, women on the contraceptive pill or hormone replacement, and people with chronic malabsorption disorders.

Zinc is present in many foods – both plant and animal, although zinc from animal foods is more readily absorbed by the body. The best sources of zinc are oysters (richest source), shellfish, red meat, poultry and cheese. Other good sources, though less easily absorbed, include legumes, whole grains, tofu, brewer's yeast, mushrooms, green beans, pumpkin and sunflower seeds. Our body does not need a large amount of zinc, but if we think we may be deficient then a dietary supplement may be required. The recommended daily allowance for healthy adults is 8–11 mg and, because zinc reduces the amount of copper our body absorbs, it is recommended that we take 2 mg of copper along with a zinc supplement. Also, because calcium reduces zinc absorption, if we are taking supplemental calcium it is important to take them at different times – perhaps calcium in the morning and zinc at midday.

Vitamin B1 (thiamine): There are eight B vitamins, all of which are needed to help the nervous system function properly and for good brain function. They are important co-factors in our stress responses and in sleep. The B vitamins are particularly important to sleep because they regulate the use of tryptophan. Vitamin B1, or thiamine, is crucial for this process and without sufficient B1 there will be decreased amounts of tryptophan. Symptoms of a B1 deficiency include fatigue, irritability, depression and abdominal discomfort. Most foods we eat contain some B1 but foods rich in this vitamin include organ meats, whole-grain or enriched cereals and rice, legumes, wheat germ, and bran. If you are healthy, but think your diet does not supply a sufficient amount of B1, a B complex vitamin supplement should be sufficient to supply the recommended daily intake (1.4 mg).

Vitamin B6 (pyridoxine): This helps convert our dietary protein to tryptophan and from tryptophan to serotonin. B6 plays an important role in our stress response and insufficient amounts of this vitamin can cause depression, irritability and insomnia. Foods high in B6 include meat, poultry, nuts, whole grains and avocado. If you think your diet is deficient in this the recommended dietary intake (2 mg) could be met by a B complex vitamin supplement.

Step 2: Changing tryptophan into serotonin

For this process to occur the body requires the minerals zinc, calcium, magnesium and iron, along with the vitamins B3, B6, C, and folate. As we have already talked about zinc and vitamin B6, we will now only discuss the other vitamins and minerals required for this step.

Calcium: Calcium is essential for converting tryptophan to serotonin. This means that not only can calcium have a calming effect (as serotonin makes us feel good) but that it also provides the serotonin that we need to produce melatonin. The important role calcium plays in good sleeping has been confirmed in the many studies that have shown that a calcium deficiency will cause increased awakenings during sleep.

If we are having trouble consolidating our sleep it may be because of insufficient calcium. This is more common in post-menopausal women; those who consume large amounts of caffeine, alcohol, or soda; and in people with chronic disorders that affect absorption. Also, because our body needs magnesium, phosphorous, and especially vitamins D and K, in order for calcium to be absorbed and used properly, a lack of any one of these may also cause a calcium deficiency.

The best way to get calcium is through food and the richest food sources of calcium are dairy products (cheese, milk and yoghurt), tofu, nuts (such as almonds, Brazil nuts and hazelnuts) and leafy green vegetables. If our diet does not contain sufficient calcium we may need to use a supplement. In healthy adults the recommended amount of calcium supplement per day is 600 mg, and it should be taken along with magnesium and vitamins D and K to increase absorption. If we take supplemental calcium we should take it in the morning hours.

Magnesium: Magnesium plays an integral role in every one of our organs and is essential to many chemical reactions throughout our body and brain. It also helps regulate calcium levels, as well as copper, zinc, potassium, vitamin D, and other important nutrients in the body. Due to its broad effects, magnesium can affect our sleep in a number of ways.

Firstly, due to its role in regulating calcium, magnesium affects our sleep regulation and when magnesium is not readily available the processes necessary for sleep cannot take place at an appropriate rate. Studies have shown that insufficient magnesium increases our wakefulness and decreases the amount of deep sleep. It has also been shown that too much magnesium will cause poor quality sleep so a *balanced* level of magnesium is important.

Secondly, magnesium is an essential element in the process of muscle relaxation. Without sufficient magnesium muscles will have trouble relaxing, causing cramps and muscle pain. This is especially so if too little magnesium is accompanied by too much calcium, as excess calcium can cause tight, contracted muscles. Increasing magnesium intake has been found to reduce the incidence of cramps and to improve the sleep of people who have Restless Legs Syndrome and fibromyalgia, presumably due to its importance in muscle relaxation.

A deficiency in magnesium can be caused by too much coffee, soda, salt or alcohol, heavy menstrual periods or excessive sweating. Prolonged stress can also lower magnesium levels. Symptoms of magnesium deficiency may include mood disturbance, such as anxiety and irritability; sleep disorders, such as insomnia and restless leg syndrome; and muscle spasm and pain.

We get magnesium from many foods and those rich in magnesium include whole grains, nuts, and green vegetables, especially green leafy vegetables. Many herbs and spices also supply magnesium including coriander, dill, celery seed, sage, dried mustard, basil, cocoa powder, cumin, tarragon and marjoram. If we think we do not get enough magnesium from our diet we may need to think about taking a magnesium supplement. The recommended dose for healthy individuals is 250 mg per day.

It's important to note that, as they work in combination with each other, magnesium and calcium should be taken together, in the morning hours. The right balance, as well as the right amount, of these minerals is required for long, consolidated and restful sleep.

Iron: Iron is an essential mineral that is required to sustain human life. It is a vital component of our red blood cells, which are responsible for delivering oxygen (and therefore energy) to all the cells of our body. Common symptoms of an iron deficiency are fatigue and tiring easily. Restless Legs Syndrome, a common cause of insomnia, is also a symptom of an iron deficiency as we saw in Chapter 11. Iron deficiency is one of the most common nutritional disorders in the world and can be caused by an iron-poor diet, an inability to absorb enough dietary iron and is sometimes a consequence of pregnancy.

Iron is present in many foods, both plant and animal, but we are more easily able to absorb the iron in animal foods. The best dietary sources of iron are organ meats, lean red meat, poultry, fish, and shellfish (particularly oysters). Other plant-based dietary sources of iron are beans and peas, legumes, nuts and seeds, whole grains, and green leafy vegetables. Because iron, in contrast to many other nutrients, is not excreted by the body, iron can build up in our system. High blood iron increases the risk for developing cardiovascular and metabolic diseases and, for this reason, we should check our blood iron level before taking a supplement. In healthy individuals recommended daily intake varies on our age and sex with males and post-menopausal women requiring much less (8 mg) than menstruating women (18 mg).

Vitamin B3 (niacin): In clinical trials niacin supplementation has been shown to improve the amount of REM sleep in normal sleepers and to increase both REM time and sleep consolidation in those with insomnia. When vitamin B3 supplementation was withdrawn from those with insomnia their sleep quality deteriorated. While it is unusual to be severely deficient in this vitamin, because bread and cereals are usually fortified with niacin, we may have a mild deficiency. Symptoms of deficiency include indigestion, fatigue, vomiting, and depression. The best food sources of vitamin B3 are found in brewer's yeast, organ meats, fish, sunflower seeds, and peanuts. If we think we may have a B3 deficiency the recommended dietary intake (18 mg) could be met by a B complex vitamin supplement.

Vitamin C (ascorbic acid): Vitamin C is essential for the manufacture of serotonin and also plays a role in decreasing our cortisol levels and supporting our stress response. If we do not have enough vitamin C we will not only have difficulty sleeping, but we may also suffer from anaemia, poor immunity, and swollen and painful joints. The best food sources of vitamin C are uncooked fruits and vegetables, which all contain some amount of vitamin C. Those richest in vitamin C are orange, kiwi fruit, grapefruit, mango, watermelon, papaya, leafy green vegetables, tomato and capsicum. Additionally some cereals and other foods and beverages are fortified with vitamin C. If we think our diet is not supplying enough vitamin C, a supplement will provide the recommended daily intake (75 mg).

Folate (folic acid): Folate is essential for the formation of serotonin and a deficiency in this vitamin can lead to sleeping difficulties. A folate deficiency also appears to play a role in Restless Legs Syndrome because when people with restless legs were given supplemental folate their symptoms improved, but there was a reappearance of the symptoms when supplementation was reduced. Dietary sources of folate include leafy green vegetables, fresh fruit, whole grains, poultry and liver. Folate content in food can be depleted by overcooking so a supplement may be necessary even in a well-balanced diet. If we think our diet is not supplying enough folate, a B complex vitamin supplement will provide the recommended daily intake (400 µg).

Step 3: From serotonin to melatonin

For this process to occur the body requires the minerals magnesium and calcium and the vitamin B5. As we have already discussed most of these vitamins and minerals we need only to find out about vitamins B5 and B12.

Vitamin B5 (pantothenic acid): This vitamin is good for relieving stress and anxiety. It plays an important role in our stress response and is involved in the regulation of cortisol (our wakeful hormone) in stressful situations. It is sometimes called the anti-stress vitamin. Symptoms of a vitamin B5 deficiency may include fatigue, insomnia, and poor mood. Foods rich in vitamin B5 include meat, eggs, vegetables and whole unprocessed grains. Be aware, however, that a lot of this vitamin will be lost if the food is refined, frozen or canned. If we think we may have a B5 deficiency the recommended dietary intake (10 mg) could be met by a B complex vitamin supplement.

Vitamin B12 (cobalamin): While vitamin B12 is not actively involved in the manufacture of serotonin or melatonin it is important in the regulation of the circadian rhythm. It is thought to do this by enhancing the light sensitivity of the body's internal clock and in a number of studies has been shown to improve both sleep and wake quality, resulting in feeling refreshed upon wakening.

As we age we lose some of our ability to absorb vitamin B12 from our foods and because there is virtually none of this vitamin in plant foods, people who follow a strict vegetarian diet may well be deficient. Insufficient amounts of this vitamin can lead to generalised body weakness, anaemia and fatigue as well as poor sleep. Good dietary sources are eggs, meat, milk and milk products, organ meats and poultry. If we think we may have deficient vitamin B12 a B vitamin complex will supply the recommended daily intake (6 µg).

The particular proteins, vitamins and minerals that we have just talked about are the basic necessities for sleep simply because our body cannot produce our sleep hormone without them. Now that we know about them we need to ensure that we have sufficient amounts of each of them in our diet. If we feel we may be deficient in any of these – and this may be due to eating the wrong foods, a problem of poor absorption, or to ageing – then we may need to consider taking vitamin or mineral supplements, which are readily available from most supermarkets and health-food stores. However, while supplements may be the answer in the short term, we should always aim to optimise what we eat to ensure that we provide the best available foods for our sleep.

The diet of normal sleepers

In a large study of over 5500 people conducted in the USA it was found that the normal sleepers (greater than 7 hours and less than 9 hours of sleep each night) ate the greatest food variety and had an increased consumption of complex carbohydrates (whole grain foods) and vitamins and minerals.

In particular the study found that normal sleepers had significantly more of the following in their diet:

- Lycopene: A cancer-fighting antioxidant found in tomatoes, watermelon and pink grapefruit.
- Vitamin C: A heart- and cancer-protective antioxidant found in uncooked fruit and vegetables.
- Selenium: An anti-inflammatory that is contained in Brazil nuts, seeds and fish.
- Theobromine: An antioxidant contained in cocoa/chocolate.
- Lauric acid: A fatty acid contained in coconut, palm oil and coconut milk. Lower amounts are also found in milk and butter.

Foods that may negatively impact sleep quality

As would be expected, and as has been experienced by many of us I am sure, what we eat can also negatively affect how we sleep. If we want to maximise our chance of consolidated sleep it is important to understand what foods may prevent us from doing so. I say 'may' because everyone is different and you may well think that some of the foods I mention here have no impact on you whatsoever. If, however, you are having trouble sleeping, you may want to consider eliminating some of these food items, and see if your sleep benefits.

Dietary fats

There is not a lot known about the effects of dietary fats on sleep but what is known indicates that if we want to sleep well we should limit our fat intake. In 2010 a study of nearly 500 women found that increased caloric and total fat intake (including saturated fat, mono-unsaturated fat and trans fat) throughout the day was associated with decreased sleep duration. This finding was further confirmed in a later study that showed that nocturnal fat consumption was associated with difficulties getting to sleep (increased sleep latency) and difficulty maintaining sleep, with a greater number of awakenings during the night in those who had a higher nocturnal fat intake.

These studies combined suggest that for deep, restful sleep we need to limit our overall intake of fats and to restrict fat intake to earlier in the day.

Dietary proteins

In the same way as there is an amino acid (tryptophan) that is essential to our sleeping pathway so too are there amino acids that are essential to our awake pathway. These amino acids are the building blocks to our 'alerting' hormones in the same way as tryptophan is the building block for melatonin. If we eat proteins containing high amounts of these particular amino acids then we may have trouble getting to sleep. Having a good understanding of what proteins are involved in making these 'alerting' hormones (and avoiding them in the evening hours) is therefore an important consideration in optimising sleep.

Glutamate (glutamic acid)

Glutamate is an amino acid and is the primary excitatory chemical of the brain. It is fundamental to the proper working of our arousal system. Glutamate is sometimes thought of as nature's brain food as it is involved in almost all aspects of normal brain function, including cognition, memory and learning.

Glutamate is present in most proteins, but it is often found in concentrated amounts in food additives and in flavour enhancers. Most of us would be familiar with the flavour enhancer MSG (monosodium glutamate), which has a high concentration of glutamate. It is often present in Asian cooking and is frequently present in salty or spicy foods. In a 2005 study researchers found that increased glutamate production resulted in increased performance in people after a sleepless night. They suggested that this was due to glutamate's ability to 'wake the brain up'. If we want to sleep well it is best to avoid foods containing concentrated amounts of glutamate at night. These foods include cheese, soy sauce, vegemite, marmite and anything containing MSG (MSG is known by a variety of names and is always present in the following ingredients: gelatin, yeast extract, soy protein and anything hydrolysed). Foods low in glutamate that are a better alternative, especially in the evening, are fruits, vegetables, potatoes, poultry and eggs.

Tyrosine

Tyrosine is another amino acid and is important for the healthy functioning of the thyroid, adrenal and pituitary glands. It is the primary building block for the body's two main stress hormones: adrenaline and noradrenaline. Tyrosine has also been found to improve cognitive function during stressful situations and dietary supplements of tyrosine are associated with improved alertness, arousal and mood.

While tyrosine, like glutamate, is important for the proper functioning of our alertness and cognitive functions, if we eat foods containing a high level of this amino acid at the wrong time of day we are increasing our chances of tossing and turning throughout the night hours. Foods containing higher amounts of tyrosine include: cheddar cheese, wheat, sesame seeds, seaweed, peanuts, and fermented meats such as salami and chorizo sausage. It is advisable to avoid these foods from the early evening onwards.

Foods containing tyramine, the breakdown product of tyrosine, should also be avoided in the evening hours if we are having difficulties sleeping. Apart from those foods already mentioned, over-ripe fruits and certain alcoholic beverages, especially Chianti, port, sherry and vermouth, contain tyramine and are therefore best avoided at night.

Stimulants

It almost goes without saying – but for the sake of completeness – stimulants will interfere with our sleep. In fact, that is exactly their purpose. As we have already looked at a variety of stimulants and their effect on the body in the previous chapter, we will not go into them again except to reiterate that caffeine (in any form), alcohol, nicotine and some drugs are all stimulants and are best to be avoided if you are having problems sleeping. Even in the absence of sleep problems they are best consumed no later than lunch-time so as to avoid having any effect on sleep.

Did you know?

If asked, I am sure many of us would nominate sugar as a food most likely to interfere with sleep and some would consider it as a stimulant due to the 'energy high' that sugar induces. But this would be wrong. Believe it or not, there is no scientific evidence that sugar causes an energy high or hyperactivity. In fact, eating sugar releases our feel-good hormone serotonin which relaxes us and makes us feel calmer – the complete opposite to the 'buzz' some people talk about.

The myth of the sugar buzz is thought to have come about near the end of World War II when all of Britain was under severe rationing, including sugar rationing. At that time the government, in an attempt to reduce sugar usage, put out propaganda saying that sugar was bad for you and caused hyperactivity in children. For some unknown reason, 70 years later, despite the fact that no controlled study has proved this effect of sugar, and numerous controlled studies have shown conclusively that sugar intake does not cause hyperactivity or mood disturbance, the myth has continued.

If you have sugar in coffee, or sugar in sweets which also have some caffeine and/or food colouring (which by contrast to sugar has been shown to affect activity and behaviour), you may well experience or observe a change in behaviour. This will not be due to the sugar content but to the additives.

So does sugar affect our sleep? The answer is yes, but in a positive way. As mentioned sugar makes us feel good because it releases serotonin, one of our happy hormones. We normally get an increase in this hormone when we do things that invigorate us and make us feel good, like exercising or walking in the sunshine. This effect of sugar is one of the reasons why if we are feeling stressed we may crave something sweet because, without thinking about it, we know subconsciously that it will make us feel good.

Serotonin is also important in helping us get to sleep. Not only does it relax us, thereby making sleep easier to come by, but serotonin is the building block for melatonin (our sleepy hormone) and if we do not have enough serotonin we cannot produce enough melatonin, making sleep elusive. So for any of us having difficulty getting to sleep a pre-bedtime snack of a glass of warm milk and a small biscuit may just do the trick.

When we think about what foods enhance, or detract from, our sleep it is important to recognise that everybody is different. For some of us, it may be that we already have a well-balanced diet that allows all the processes of sleep to occur and all the hormones of sleep to be manufactured. It may be that our difficulty with sleep has little to do with diet, but is the result of an undiagnosed sleep disorder or bad sleep habits. For others, you may now realise that your diet has been working against you, preventing good sleep, and it is time to ensure that your diet contains all the correct foods, minerals and vitamins in the right amount.

Optimising your diet for good sleep is a good place to start but keep in mind that the causes of poor sleep can be multi-factorial. It may be that your sleep difficulties are due to a combination of poor diet *and* poor sleep habits, or poor diet *and* a sleep disorder. It is only by examining and eliminating each of these potential causes that you will be guaranteed deep, restful sleep.

Putting it all together

A diet good for all aspects of our sleep is based on fresh whole foods, along with:

1. Good fat: Foods which have a high content of mono- or poly-unsaturated fats are better than those with saturated or trans fats. The good fat foods are nuts, seeds, fish, skinless poultry and olive, canola or sunflower oils. These healthy fats are also good sources of essential vitamins and trace minerals required for sleep (unlike ice-cream).
2. Good protein: Animal and plant protein are both good for us. Some animal protein, like red meat, has a high amount of saturated fats, which isn't healthy, so a better animal protein choice is fish or poultry. Good vegetable sources are beans, nuts, and whole grains, all of which provide us with essential vitamins and minerals.
3. Good carbohydrate: The best sources of carbohydrates are whole grains (the less processed the better) and unprocessed whole fruit and vegetables, especially leafy green vegetables, which provide a good source of vitamins and trace minerals. Refined carbohydrates, such as white bread, white rice, cakes, soft drink and fruit juice, contain minimal fibre and a high amount of simple sugars, which provide little nutritional content but high calorie content. These types of carbohydrates do not assist our sleep in any way.

If you feel that despite eating a fresh whole food diet you may still be deficient in some of the vitamins and trace minerals it is important that you supplement your diet appropriately.

What to eat at night

Foods that are good for sleep contain tryptophan, which helps produce serotonin (our feel-good hormone) and melatonin (our sleep hormone). By ensuring that we eat foods high in tryptophan in the evening hours we are giving ourselves the best chance of consolidated sleep. There are many foods that contain a good amount of tryptophan including the ones listed below:

- poultry (skinless)
- leafy green vegetables
- mushrooms
- nuts such as hazelnuts and almonds (good for the occasional evening snack when hungry)
- milk

What not to eat at night

Foods that should be avoided at night are those that work to wake us up. These foods often contain tyrosine, tyramine or glutamate, all of which stimulate our awake hormones. Eating these foods late at night will often result in disturbed sleep and an over-active mind, sometimes causing nightmares. These foods include:

- aged and processed meat
- cheese
- soy beans and soy products
- over-ripe fruit
- many types of spicy foods as they contain MSG (monosodium glutamate)

It is also important to avoid known stimulants like caffeine and alcohol.

Chapter 17

Women and sleep

THERE ARE SIGNIFICANT PHYSIOLOGICAL DIFFERENCES **between men and women, and it is just beginning to be recognised that a woman's sexual hormones play a significant role in her ability to manage good sleep.**

Vicki's story

All her life Vicki had slept exceptionally well. She clearly remembered the time when she would regularly go to sleep around 10.30 pm sleeping soundly until about 7 am the following day, when she would get up feeling refreshed and ready to greet the day. Recently this had all changed and Vicki had been having disturbed sleep for at least the past year. She knew the reason for her problem but did not know what to do about it.

Vicki was 52 years old and experiencing hot flushes. She was having them both day and night but they were particularly noticeable at night when they would wake her up several times, leaving her quite agitated. Once the hot flush passed she found it difficult to get back to sleep and, as a result, she was getting much less sleep than she needed, which left her feeling tired and unmotivated. When she spoke to her doctor about the problem he wanted to prescribe antidepressants but Vicki didn't think that she was actually depressed – rather she was just really tired and needed her old sleeping pattern back.

She discussed hormone replacement therapy with her doctor, but given her family history of breast cancer she decided she wasn't the ideal candidate for it. She was starting to reconsider her decision about antidepressants and was also contemplating sleeping tablets, but when she had used these in the past they made her feel 'foggy' the next day, so she was searching for a natural solution to the problem.

Vicki's problem is extremely common and for many women menopause is one of the times that they can encounter serious sleep problems. I say 'one of the times' for a very good reason.

Up until the last 10 years almost nothing was known about the effect of the hormones oestrogen and progesterone on sleep or what effects changing levels of these hormones could have on women. In the past almost all research had focused on the mood changes women experienced at these times without considering that some of these mood changes may be partially the result of a problem with sleep. As a result, some women today are being treated for depression and taking antidepressant medication without any investigation into whether the depression is a consequence of the sleeplessness caused by the changes in their sexual hormone levels.

It is interesting that the sleep consequences of fluctuating sexual hormones have not been investigated until recently, especially as it has been known for some time that there are definite sex differences in sleep–wake patterns of males and females. Throughout their lives females require more sleep than males – on average they need about 20 minutes more sleep than their male counterparts. Up until puberty girls are better sleepers and get more sleep but, with the onset of puberty, adolescent women may start to experience insomnia and difficulty with sleep onset. These sleep problems persist in adulthood and women have an increased risk for insomnia and report more sleep difficulties than men.

The differences in how men and women sleep is important information and essential for all women who want to get deep, restful sleep. It is important for women to understand that their hormones can significantly negatively impact their sleep and that this impact can occur from the onset of puberty, throughout pregnancy and breastfeeding, and through and beyond menopause. It is also critical to understand that these sleep difficulties can be additional to any other underlying sleep disorder that we have already learned about in this book. So in this chapter I am going to discuss the various stages of womanhood and the potential impact these have on the ability to achieve deep, restful sleep, as well as possible solutions to these issues.

Sleep and the menstrual cycle

To begin with we are going to look at how the menstrual cycle can affect women's sleep. Understanding what is happening during this time and recognising any connections between poor sleep and where a woman is at in her monthly cycle enables her to implement practices that can, to a degree, counteract these negative effects and allow her to get good sleep no matter what the time of the month.

Before I start investigating this it is worth quickly summarising the cycle of menstruation and what happens with oestrogen and progesterone during this time. In the normal cycle of 28 days, the first day of bleeding is referred to as day 1. There are two phases in the cycle: phase 1 occurs before ovulation (which happens around day 14) and is called the follicular phase, because it is during this time that the follicle (egg) grows. The follicular phase is associated with an increasing level of oestrogen, which peaks just before ovulation. Following ovulation there is a sudden decline in oestrogen and a progressively increasing level of progesterone. This second, post-ovulation phase is referred to as the luteal phase. Approximately 14 days after ovulation, if there is no implantation of a fertilised egg, both progesterone and oestrogen levels drop sharply bringing on the start of bleeding. These changes in hormone levels throughout the monthly cycle are illustrated in the following diagram. Ovulatory cycles are typically between 25 and 35 days and it is during the last week of the cycle, and during the first few days of bleeding when oestrogen and progesterone levels are dropping, that women experience their most negative menstrual symptoms.

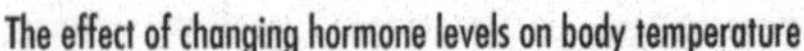

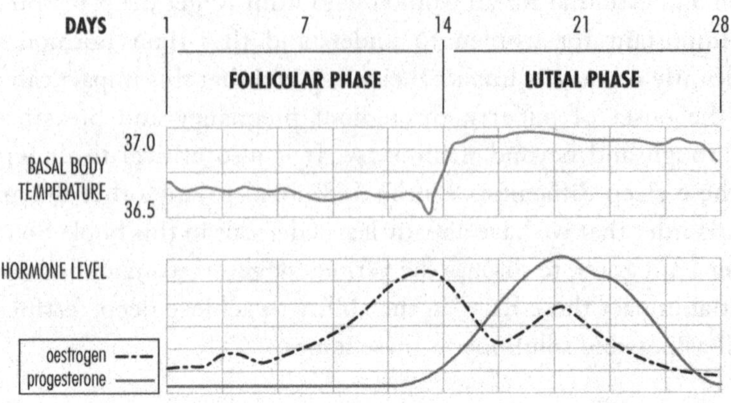

One of the most important changes brought about by the menstrual cycle is that the basal body temperature is higher in the luteal phase than it is in the follicular phase (when oestrogen dominates). In Chapter 3, we learned that our core body temperature fluctuates throughout the day and, although it only fluctuates by 1°C (between 36°C and 37°C), it is the nightly fall in temperature that greatly assists our ability to initiate sleep. If we look at the diagram above we can see that there is an increase in temperature of between 0.4°C and 0.6°C in the second phase of the menstrual cycle. Even though this is only a small increase and not something women would usually notice, it is sufficient to blunt the fall in temperature that we rely upon to help initiate sleep as the basal body temperature is only able to drop by 0.6°C (and perhaps only 0.4°C). For some women this blunted temperature decline causes a delay in their sleep cycle, such that even though they may go to bed at the same time as in the first phase of their cycle they will have difficulty getting to sleep (sleep-onset insomnia). As a consequence these women will suffer some degree of sleep deprivation in the second phase of their cycle and may experience fatigue and poor mood state. While it is generally not recognised, lack of sleep also decreases the ability to withstand pain and when sleep deprived we feel pain more keenly, which may account to some degree as to why so many women experience severe pain at menstruation.

It has also been recently discovered that some women have decreased melatonin levels in the second phase compared to the first, which can make sleep onset and sleep maintenance difficult. When we add decreased melatonin with the blunted temperature decline we can begin to understand why some women have significant problems with their sleep during the second phase of their cycle. Indeed, it is not at all surprising that for the 20–25% of women who have menstrual-related problems, such as mood disorders or cramping pain, there is a three-fold increase in insomnia and excessive daytime sleepiness in the week preceding the start of menstruation.

Emerging research indicates that there is a strong connection between the phases of the menstrual cycle, sleep disturbances and complaints of menstrual symptoms. Knowing this allows us to develop strategies that can go some way to improving these symptoms.

The first thing that must be done is to work out whether any symptoms suffered are a consequence of the menstrual cycle. This is easily done by filling out the sleep and mood diary at the end of this chapter for two complete menstrual cycles. If the mood and fatigue symptoms fluctuate along with the cycle then it is clear that they are a result of hormone fluctuations. If you detect cyclical symptoms then you may benefit from implementing the following 11 strategies:

1. Continue to record your cycle along with your mood and level of fatigue so that you become familiar with your body's rhythm. This knowledge will allow you to anticipate and prepare for any mood or sleep disturbance.
2. Do not dismiss your feelings of fatigue and do not try to battle through them. Although it is not widely acknowledged it needs to be recognised that progesterone has a soporific effect (it induces sleep) and the increase of this hormone in the second part of the cycle frequently results in very real feelings of increased sleepiness. If you experience increased fatigue and daytime sleepiness as you get closer to menstruation it is important to recognise the reason for this and respond to your body's signals. It is especially important in the week leading up to menstruation to accept the greater requirement for sleep and increase your sleep time. While this may be annoying initially it will pay off as you will no longer suffer the fatigue and brain 'fogginess' that you may previously have felt in the week leading up to the start of bleeding.

3. Have your doctor check your iron and ferritin levels. If they are low or on the lower side of normal then you might benefit from taking a dietary supplement. As we saw earlier in Chapter 11 restless legs, which are disruptive to sleep, can be caused by reduced iron levels, so it is a good idea to consider this.
4. Try supplementing your diet with calcium, magnesium and L-tryptophan, all of which have been shown to have a positive effect in alleviating effects of premenstrual syndrome.
5. Consider using a melatonin supplement in the second phase of your cycle. Some women find that this may be effective in consolidating sleep. Numerous clinical trials have also shown Chasteberry (*Vitex agnus-castus*) to be effective at alleviating menstrual symptoms, probably due to its enhancement of serotonin (our relaxing hormone and the precursor to melatonin).
6. Try to schedule a 20-minute afternoon nap around the time of your afternoon dip in alertness (see Chapter 3) whenever possible in the week before menstruation and for the first few days of bleeding. This will decrease your feelings of tiredness but not interfere with your night-time sleep.
7. Be diligent with your sleep practices in the second phase of your cycle and do not have caffeine after midday.
8. Minimise exposure to light after 8 pm in the second phase and switch off all technology one hour before bed to allow melatonin production.
9. Have a warm to hot shower just before bedtime. After the shower the skin temperature decreases and will enhance the natural decrease in temperature thereby improving your ability to get to sleep.
10. Take an analgesic for pain relief if you suffer from pain or cramping – paracetamol or ibuprofen are effective at relieving menstrual pain and can improve sleep.
11. If you are having trouble getting to sleep read Chapter 8 and try implementing the steps outlined there, such as CBT and staying in bed only when sleepy. Similarly if you are having

trouble staying asleep and are experiencing prolonged night-time wake periods, reread Chapter 9 and implement the steps outlined there.

What if my symptoms don't change?

If, after filling in the sleep and mood diary for two complete cycles, it is clear that your mood and sleep symptoms are with you all the time and the severity does not ebb and flow then it may be that you have an undiagnosed sleep disorder or one of the types of insomnias that we have discussed. In this case you may need to reread some of the information already given in other chapters. If your problems with sleep still do not resolve it is important to discuss them with your doctor.

Diligently implementing these strategies and being aware of where you are at in your cycle will facilitate deep, restful sleep all month long. If, however, after 2 months you have not experienced substantial improvements in symptoms then it is important that you speak with your doctor as there are some medications that may improve the more severe menstrual symptoms, but they do need to be taken under medical supervision. Always be aware though that how a woman sleeps throughout her monthly cycle is an important consideration in treating any menstrual symptoms.

Polycystic Ovary Syndrome (PCOS)

Polycystic Ovary Syndrome (PCOS) affects between 4–12% of women of reproductive age. Typically they present with irregular cycles, excess of male hormone (evident as excessive hairiness) and 50% are obese. Due to the excess male hormone and the excess weight, women with PCOS are 30 times more likely to have sleep apnoea than other women of the same age and weight. In Chapter 12 we discussed sleep apnoea and how it can be a cause of insomnia – whether it be sleep onset, sleep maintenance or early morning wakening. If you think you may have PCOS and sleep apnoea it is important that this is diagnosed as soon as possible and treated. As mentioned before, CPAP is an effective treatment and will lead to an almost immediate improvement in mood and fatigue symptoms.

Sleep and pregnancy

Many women experience numerous sleep disturbances for the first time during pregnancy. This is a period of great hormonal and physical change and these changes can cause significant disruption to sleep quality resulting in increased fatigue and daytime sleepiness as well as, at times, considerable distress. At some stage during pregnancy the vast majority of women (84%) report having one or more symptom of insomnia at least a few nights a week and almost a third of women report that they never or rarely get a good night's sleep during pregnancy. Some of the more common sleep problems during pregnancy include poor sleep quality, difficulty getting to sleep or staying asleep, feeling unrefreshed in the morning, daytime fatigue, irritability and lack of concentration.

Many women just accept these sleep disruptions, considering them to be a fact of life. It is now being more and more recognised that good quality sleep is a necessity for good maternal health, foetal development and optimal pregnancy outcomes. Sleep's role in a smooth transition from pregnancy to early motherhood is also now being acknowledged. It is therefore important if you are pregnant or contemplating pregnancy to be aware of the sort of sleep disruptions you may encounter during pregnancy and how best to manage these. As the nature of sleep disturbances change throughout the pregnancy the details of these are presented according to the stage of pregnancy.

First trimester

For many, fatigue is one of the first symptoms of pregnancy. About 40% of women experience this and it is commonly due to the increased level of progesterone – which increases our need for sleep. Increased fatigue may also be a result of pre-pregnancy low levels of iron or ferritin.

Sleep disruptions are also common in the first trimester due to some of the features of early pregnancy, including increased need to urinate, backache, heartburn, vomiting and nausea, which only serve to add to feelings of tiredness.

Early pregnancy can also be a time of anxiety, especially in the case of an unplanned pregnancy, and this can cause significant sleep disruption.

There are some strategies that can be implemented to reduce some of these negative side effects:

1. If possible, prior to pregnancy ensure that your folate, iron and ferritin levels are well within normal range. If these are not within normal range speak with your doctor about supplementing your diet.
2. Recognise that it is normal to be tired during this time and accept it. Make sleep a priority and plan a regular sleep–wake schedule. If necessary, add 20-minute naps during the day.
3. Drink lots of fluids during the day but restrict fluids before bedtime to reduce nocturnal urination.
4. Eat a balanced diet providing magnesium, potassium, calcium and vitamin C (to increase folate absorption from food).
5. If heartburn is disrupting your sleep, refrain from spicy or acidic food, and eat only a small meal at night at least 3 hours before bedtime. Elevating the head of the bed may also relieve symptoms.
6. Exercise regularly every day for at least 30 minutes as this will reduce any stress and improve your ability to maintain sleep.
7. Be diligent with good sleep practices and ensure that your bedroom is dark, cool and comfortable. Use a night light in the bathroom to decrease exposure to light which may affect melatonin secretion.
8. Do a relaxation exercise before bedtime as this will help consolidate sleep.
9. If you are having anxious thoughts about the pregnancy practise some CBT (see Chapter 7).

Implementing these strategies may not completely solve all your sleep problems but they should improve them to some extent. Importantly, they form a solid foundation for achieving deep, restful sleep for the remainder of the pregnancy.

Second trimester

The good news is that during the second trimester sleep disruptions do improve due to the body's gradual habituation to the hormonal changes. Feelings of nausea, daytime sleepiness and urination frequency decrease. As a result, women's energy levels and feelings of well-being mostly increase during this time. Towards the end of this trimester, however, sleep again begins to be disrupted and this can be due to a variety of reasons:

- Due to the increasing size of the foetus, foetal movements are felt more keenly, heartburn can become problematic and there is a return of the need for increased urination, all of which can cause multiple nocturnal awakenings and result in sleep fragmentation.
- Many women begin to suffer leg cramps. While this may occur in the first 3 months it is much more common in the second trimester with nearly 60% of women experiencing them.
- During this time 20% of women may develop Restless Legs Syndrome (RLS), which is discussed in Chapter 11. Luckily it generally resolves after delivery. Unluckily though, it is often not recognised and, for many women, RLS causes significant sleep disruption and all the negative consequences of sleep deprivation.
- Many women may develop shortness of breath along with snoring at some time during this trimester that may disturb sleep. As the pregnancy progresses there is an increased risk of developing sleep apnoea especially in obese women (sleep apnoea during pregnancy is discussed in more detail below).

Managing sleep during this trimester involves maintaining all the sleep strategies implemented in the first trimester while adding in these extra practices:

1. If heartburn continues to disrupt sleep, despite following the strategies suggested for the first trimester, consult your doctor about antacid therapy.
2. If you are experiencing leg cramping, speak with your doctor about supplementing your diet with magnesium lactate or

magnesium citrate, both of which have been shown to alleviate this problem. Reducing phosphorus-containing substances, like milk and meat, as well as nightly stretching and massage before bedtime have also been shown to give various levels of relief.

3. The use of pregnancy support pillows between the knees and under the abdomen may improve cramping and increase sleeping comfort.
4. RLS is more prevalent in women who have deficient or low (but within normal) levels of iron and folate. Levels of haemoglobin, ferritin and vitamin B12 start to fall in the second half of pregnancy due to the growing needs of the foetus. It is important that these levels are monitored and, if low, you should consult your doctor about supplementation. RLS is also improved by exercise so make sure you continue with the 30 minutes of daily exercise that you started in the first trimester.
5. Snoring may prevent consolidated sleep and can be improved by a variety of practices.
   (a) Try sleeping in a semi-upright position – this will reduce snoring as well as heartburn.
   (b) As sleeping on your back increases the likelihood of snoring and if sleeping semi-upright is not for you, try sleeping on your left side. This will improve blood flow to the foetus as well as the mother's body.
   (c) Relieve any nasal congestion with saline nasal washes or nasal dilators, and avoid active and passive smoking and alcohol.
   (d) As snoring in this trimester increases the likelihood of sleep apnoea it is important if you are overweight to proactively minimise weight gain. This is your best protection to prevent the development of sleep apnoea.

Third trimester

For all sorts of reasons the third trimester is the most challenging for achieving good sleep. During this time the majority of women report restless sleep and nearly all report multiple nocturnal awakenings due to the continuation of symptoms that began emerging towards the end of the second trimester, like frequent urination, backache, leg cramp and so on. If you have been diligent in implementing the strategies suggested up to this point you will be in a good position to cope with these challenges.

Along with the worsening of physical symptoms women can also suffer sleep loss to other factors, including:

- Dreaming vividly.
- Concerns about pregnancy outcomes make sleep onset and maintenance difficult for some women.
- Heightened feelings of anxiety that may be caused by the development of any pregnancy complications, such as gestational diabetes and hypertension, will also heighten any anxiety already being felt.
- Snoring may increase in loudness and frequency and can be an indicator of the development of sleep apnoea (especially if overweight or obese pre-pregnancy). If you snore loudly, have pauses in breathing or wake up gasping you need to consult your doctor about the possibility of sleep apnoea. It is slowly being recognised that this can be a serious condition in pregnancy and emerging research is indicating that sleep apnoea is significantly associated with, and exacerbates, gestational hypertension, gestational diabetes and pre-eclampsia.

Sleep apnoea has been discussed in detail in Chapter 12 and, as explained in that chapter, every time there is an apnoea there is a decrease in the amount of oxygen in the blood (as the person has effectively stopped breathing). The oxygen level only normalises once breathing recommences when the person arouses and effectively reopens their airway. While this has serious consequences for the mother, increasing her risk of developing gestational diabetes, gestational hypertension and pre-eclampsia, some research indicates that the decreases in oxygen and the sleep fragmentation also have devastating effects on the developing foetus. Untreated sleep apnoea increases the risk of premature delivery, unplanned caesareans, low birth weight and low Apgar scores.

Managing good sleep in the third trimester can sometimes be difficult and so it is important that all the sleep strategies outlined so far are implemented and maintained throughout the course of the pregnancy.

In this last trimester it is also important to:

1. Manage increasing pain and discomfort with massage, local heat and pillow support.
2. Practise relaxation techniques – in particular breathing techniques (see Chapter 6) – to reduce the contractions and any muscle tension brought on by anxiety.
3. If you are having difficulties getting to sleep and/or staying asleep try practising CBT or some of the other techniques (like staying in bed only when sleepy) outlined in chapters 8 and 9.
4. Continue to factor naps into your day – although, if you are having trouble sleeping at night make sure that these are only for about 20 minutes, otherwise you may find your night-time sleep worsening.
5. Minimise weight gain in this trimester if you are overweight as it will improve the quality of sleep and reduce snoring, as well as the risk of sleep apnoea.
6. Consult your doctor if you think you may have sleep apnoea. Studies have shown that treating sleep apnoea with CPAP normalises foetal outcomes and improves maternal health.

For all of us, insufficient or poor quality sleep at any time is detrimental to our mood state and emotional sensitivity and can trigger physical and psychological stress or depression. This is particularly so in pregnancy. Being able to get deep, restful sleep throughout this entire period can make the world of difference to the experience of pregnancy. Crucially it has been found that women with sleep disruption during late pregnancy are at higher risk of emotional disturbance in the first few weeks after delivery than women who reported better sleep. For both mother and baby getting sleep right during pregnancy is essential for optimal outcomes and it is important that strategies are put in place from even before pregnancy to ensure that deep, restful sleep can happen.

Sleep and the post-partum period

Sleeping in pregnancy is just the start of what can be a continuous challenge to achieve the sleep required after the birth of the baby. The experience of extreme tiredness for new mothers is almost universal during the post-partum period (generally defined as from delivery until about 6 months post-delivery). In this time the new mother experiences significant physiological, emotional and sociological changes and, if she is not getting adequate sleep, she is not well placed to manage these changes. That is not to say that fathers do not undergo substantial changes in their lives as well, but the woman experiences these changes after 9 months of pregnancy, which may have left her feeling depleted and sleep deprived even before the birth. She also has the additional bodily changes post-birth to deal with.

In the following section I will describe what we currently know about post-partum sleep and provide strategies that may be effective in reducing some of the negative impacts a newborn baby can have on parental sleep.

While the post-partum period is defined as the time between delivery until around 6 months post-delivery it is often divided into 3 stages: Stage 1 is the first 48 hours post-delivery, Stage 2 is from 2 days to 6 weeks, and Stage 3 is from 6 weeks to 6 months. In each stage feelings of fatigue and sleep can be differentially affected.

In Stage 1 the abrupt drop in hormone levels can affect the new mother's sleep as much as the 24-hour care she needs to provide the newborn. Melatonin levels can also be affected due to the increased light exposure at night that she encounters in the hospital nursery and the decreased light exposure during the day as a consequence of restricted activity in the outside environment. In this first 48-hour period maternal sleep is poor, especially if there has been a night labour. Research has found that night labour is linked to the development of post-partum depression in the first weeks post birth.

In stage 2, new mothers are also at risk of anaemia (due to the increased demands of the pregnancy and blood loss during the birth) and infection (endometriosis, urinary tract infection and mastitis). During the second post-partum stage if the mother is experiencing high levels of fatigue these possibilities need to be assessed.

To breastfeed or not?

At around the 6 week point (Stage 3) many women are tempted to give up breastfeeding in the hope that feeding with formula will satisfy the baby more, allowing for longer sleeping periods during the night. Research has not borne out this hope. In the first few weeks, self-reported sleep disturbance and perception of fatigue do not differ between mothers who breastfeed and mothers who formula-feed, but by 3 months breastfed babies sleep on average 45 minutes more per night than formula-fed infants.

Apart from these issues though, and as would be expected, the overriding cause of fatigue in the post-partum period is the sleeplessness caused by the newborn baby's numerous nocturnal awakenings, contributing to severely disrupted sleep for both the mother and father. As a result, fatigue is often a major issue at this time, significantly impairing a parent's ability to enjoy the first few months of their baby's life. Up to 60% of all new mothers experience post-natal blues within the first 2 weeks. While this is mostly short-lived, up to 15% of women will go on to develop a full-blown depression – post-partum depression – which for many is extremely debilitating. Over the years the cause of this depression has proven difficult to elucidate and the likely culprits, such as difficulties with delivery, overly high expectations of motherhood, and the dramatic drop in hormone levels, have not been found to be directly linked to it.

The one variable that has been traditionally overlooked, but is likely to play a significant role, is the sleep deprivation and disrupted sleep cycles that these women experience. As mentioned earlier, being in labour during the night is associated with a higher incidence of post-natal blues. While it has always been considered that maternal depression was a result of 'hormones', it has been shown recently that having a negative mood state is more directly associated with the frequency of nightly awakenings than varying hormone levels.

Additionally, many mothers who develop the more serious post-partum depression have been shown to have significantly different sleep patterns than their non-depressed counterparts. Mothers with major depressive symptoms at 4 and 8 weeks after delivery are more likely to report having less than 6 hours' sleep in a 24-hour period in the previous week and being awakened by their baby three or more times during the hours of 10 pm to 6 am.

It is also now recognised that some infant sleep problems are associated with poor general health in mothers and fathers. In mothers with no past history of depression, infant sleep problems increased the risk of the mother presenting with severe psychological distress.

These results should not surprise us. Throughout this book we have learned the incredible effect sleep has on our mood and so it is almost to be expected that new mothers who suffer chronic sleep deprivation and sleep disruption may experience depression. The pity of it all is that it has taken such a long time to be recognised. Now that we know this is a significant issue it is essential that new parents, and care-givers, are educated as to how they can optimise sleep during this time and beyond.

From the few studies that have been done it appears that the best approach is two-pronged. Firstly, the parents need to be educated about sleep: what it is and how to manage it. Secondly, they need to address, as early as possible, any problems with their infant's sleep. The following are some strategies that may be helpful in getting your sleep and your baby's back on track.

Establishing a circadian rhythm

When they are first born infants have no circadian rhythm which means they can (and do) wake at any time during the 24-hour period, and up until about 15 weeks of age the majority of babies do not have a day/night pattern of sleeping. After this time a circadian pattern of sleeping starts to emerge and by around 17 weeks some babies will have developed a consolidated sleeping period during the dark hours. It is not until around 22–26 weeks, however, that a clear pattern of sleep between about 8 pm to 6 am is present in the majority of infants.

This is important information for a new parent. Firstly, it may reassure them that what their baby is doing is completely normal and allows them to have realistic expectations for what is possible with their baby's sleep in this early period.

Secondly, by understanding the importance of establishing a circadian rhythm, parents can begin to entrain their baby's rhythm to a pattern of day/night as early as possible. Entraining the baby's circadian rhythm is done in the same way as is done in adults:

- As exposure to light is the biggest determinant of circadian pattern, parents need to ensure that the baby is exposed to light in the morning and dim light in the evening. At night, always use a dim night light so that exposure to light at this time is limited.
- The baby's activity schedule needs to be as regular as possible with restricted play in the evening hours.
- Feeding also needs to be regular, and after 3 months of age the time between feeds should be extended in the night hours.
- When the baby awakes at night, any stimulation needs to be kept to a minimum.

Implementing these practices optimises the chances of your baby's biological clock becoming in tune with the 24-hour day as early as possible. However, be sure to keep expectations realistic and keep in mind that establishing a day/night sleeping pattern can take up to 6 months.

Responding to crying

By 6 months of age the majority of babies will have established a circadian rhythm so that most of their sleep is in the night hours. While this is usually great news for parents, it isn't so great if the child continually wakes throughout this period and needs parental attention to get back to sleep. To minimise the risk of this happening, and to help the baby self-settle, parents should respond only if the infant is genuinely crying (as opposed to fussing or fretting).

In a trial involving 260 babies, the parents of 130 babies were recommended to leave their infant to settle for 5 minutes before responding to the infant's cries, and to extend this response time by 5 minutes for each subsequent visit. At 12 weeks, those babies were twice as likely to have at least 15 hours of sleep per 24 hours compared to the 130 babies whose parents did not implement this practice.

Of course, while parents may do all that is possible to assist their baby to sleep through the night and to develop a night-time pattern of sleeping, it will take time.

Other strategies

A few other strategies that parents can follow that may help:

1. If you have had a night labour be aware of the research showing the link between this and the development of the post-natal blues. As much as is practical, plan to catch up on the lost sleep so that by the time you leave hospital you are better rested.
2. Follow good sleep practices (Chapter 15) and be careful about maintaining your own circadian rhythm. During the baby's early weeks if parents are not careful they will disrupt their melatonin secretion by exposure to light at night – so always be careful not to turn on bright lights or do anything that alerts your mind during the night hours. The common advice given to mothers at this time (sleep when the baby sleeps) is counterintuitive when it comes to maintaining a good circadian rhythm. If possible practise the habit of napping when the baby sleeps (Chapter 3) so that after 20–25 minutes of sleeping you feel refreshed and able to continue with the day without interfering with your ability to get to sleep or stay asleep that night.
3. Be aware of how much sleep you are getting. If you are not getting enough, do something about it. Sometimes one parent is unaware of how much sleep the other parent is not getting. It is a good idea to keep a sleep diary and have a sleep plan to ensure both parents get enough sleep. This means that if the mother has had less than 6 hours' sleep 2 nights in a row, then on the third night she needs to get at least 8 hours' uninterrupted sleep. If the baby is being breastfed this will require the mother to express enough milk for the night-time feeds. Doing this allows for both parents to be adequately, although not ideally, rested.

Something to remember

Whether the baby sleeps in the same room as you or in another room is a personal choice. No matter what the choice, co-sleeping is not recommended. Bed sharing is one of the biggest risk factors for sudden infant death syndrome (SIDS) so regardless of how tired you are, after feeding or settling your baby, you need to put your baby back in their own crib to sleep.

Recognising the importance of sleep during pregnancy and the post-partum period is fundamental. Even though it is common opinion that sleep disappears the moment the baby appears, it does not have to be so. With good planning, this time of your life does not have to be one of exhaustion and bags under the eyes. Numerous studies have shown that parents educated about their sleep and their baby's sleep, and who are focused on developing healthy infant sleep patterns, get more sleep, feel more competent, are less stressed and have greater marital satisfaction than those who do not actively implement such practices.

Sleep and menopause

Insomnia and fatigue are among the most common health complaints of perimenopausal and post-menopausal women. It is estimated that about 50% of women between 40–60 years of age experience trouble sleeping, and perimenopausal and post-menopausal women are twice as likely to be dissatisfied with their sleep as premenopausal women. While it is assumed by many that this is a direct consequence of menopause this is not always so. In a number of cases the sleep disturbance may be related to conditions associated with ageing such as obesity, chronic illness and pain, rather than menopause.

While keeping this in mind, and recognising the processes of ageing for women in mid-life, there are two common clinical conditions that are experienced at this time that greatly affect the quality of sleep: sleep apnoea and hot flushes.

Sleep apnoea

Menopause is a recognised risk factor for the development of sleep apnoea (see Chapter 12). The reasons for this are not completely clear, except that many women at this time put on weight. Recent reports indicate that in Australia about 32% of women in this age group are obese and about 33% are overweight and this weight gain may be a primary risk factor for the development of sleep apnoea. Another reason may be that at this time women lose the protection of the hormone progesterone, which is a respiratory stimulant. Regardless of the reasons for the increase in the incidence of sleep apnoea at this time, its consequences can be severe – it increases the risk of depression, heart disease and metabolic dysfunction as well as causing extreme fatigue and insomnia.

Despite the fact that research clearly shows that post-menopausal women are more than four times more likely to have severe sleep apnoea than their premenopausal counterparts it is often undiagnosed or misdiagnosed. A woman presenting to her doctor at this time with fatigue, insomnia and poor mood state can, because of her presenting symptoms, be misdiagnosed with depression consequent to the onset of menopause with sometimes little consideration given to the possibility of a sleep disorder such as sleep apnoea.

So, if you are in mid-life, have recently gained a few kilos and snore it is important that you consult your doctor about the possibility of sleep apnoea. If you are diagnosed with sleep apnoea then by following the steps set out in Chapter 12 you will be able to manage it easily and discover a new lease on life.

Hot flushes and night sweats

Hot flushes are probably the most recognised of all menopausal symptoms. They are best described as episodic sensations of heat, intense sweating and flushing that affect the face and chest and which are often accompanied by palpitations and anxiety. They can last from 3–10 minutes with varied frequency – some women experience hot flushes hourly or daily, whereas for others they may occur only occasionally.

Did you know?

The exact reason why hot flushes occur is still not completely understood. Clearly they are related to changing levels of oestrogen but this is not the only factor as not all women experience hot flushes.

All of us, men and women both, can at any time in our life experience a hot flush (the telltale blush, or the feeling of heat around the neck) when, for example, we are extremely stressed or embarrassed. Understanding why and how this happens is critical to our understanding of hot flushes.

For our body to be able to fight any stress it confronts, whether it be the stress of giving a talk to a full auditorium or the stress caused by an impending attack, it needs energy. The only way the body can provide this extra energy is to increase the rate at which we burn our fuel. In other words: by increasing our metabolic rate. As soon as our metabolic rate increases, though, so too does our body temperature and the typical sign of this is the flushed or sweaty face that we may encounter when we are embarrassed by some situation or when we run for the bus.

This increase in metabolic rate is brought about by the production of the stress hormones adrenaline and noradrenalin. How much of these hormones we produce and how much our body temperature increases depends on the intensity and duration of the stress. Ordinarily when we are faced by a minor stress like, say, a traffic jam, only small amounts of these hormones will be produced and so our body temperature will not increase very much.

Mostly in these minor-stress circumstances we do not notice the slight increase in body temperature because we have a temperature zone wherein slight changes in temperature do not cause a physical response. This zone is referred to as our thermo-neutral zone and it allows for body temperature to fluctuate by as much as +0.4°C or –0.4°C without us feeling any physical consequences.

Our body creates this thermo-neutral zone by cleverly using oestrogen to dampen the effect of noradrenaline, the hormone primarily responsible for the increase in temperature. In other words oestrogen can be thought of as a kind of temperature shield and we can experience a +0.4°C or -0.4°C change in temperature without it being felt by the rest of the body. Beyond this, though, the temperature-shield effect of oestrogen disappears and the body will begin to respond either by shivering or sweating.

At menopause, however, women stop producing oestrogen and therefore no longer have this temperature shield. This means that for the vast majority of peri-menopausal and menopausal women the thermo-neutral zone is substantially narrowed (and even for some it becomes non-existent) such that any minor change in temperature, even +0.1°C or –0.1°C will induce a bodily response such as sweating and facial flushing or shivering.

It is thought that it is the *changing* levels of oestrogen that cause this rather than little or no oestrogen, as most women only experience them for one or two years until their oestrogen level stabilises, and children and men don't experience them.

Hot flushes are a common complaint of menopause with up to 75% of women experiencing them at some stage. They can cause considerable sleep disruption and it has been shown they decrease sleep efficiency, increase nightly awakenings and result in more sleep state changes. In one study assessing the effects of hot flushes it was found that of 47 objectively measured hot flushes, 45 were associated with an awakening that occurred within 5 minutes before or after the flush.

While the constant awakenings due to hot flushes would be sufficient in themselves to cause considerable sleep disturbances and unrefreshing sleep, the problem is compounded considerably because when a woman is wakened later in the sleep period – when her sleep drive has significantly decreased (and as a consequence is no longer as tired as when she first went to sleep) – she may find it harder to get straight back to sleep. Traditionally the treatment of choice for women experiencing significant discomfort and sleep deprivation was hormone replacement therapy (HRT). There is, however, controversy about the advisability of using this long term and women are now being advised to use this for the shortest term possible.

The good news is that now more is known about some of the causes of hot flushes (see box above) more treatments are being trialled with varying degrees of success. There are a number of pharmacological therapies available including certain types of antidepressants (SSRIs), which need to be taken under the advice of a physician. As a first line of defence it may be advisable to try complementary and alternative therapies, along with behavioural therapies and lifestyle modifications, which have been shown to be effective for some women.

Complementary medicines

There are numerous complementary medicines that have been explored for the treatment of hot flushes. These include black cohosh, vitamin E, evening primrose oil, dong quai, ginseng and wild yam. There is, however, little scientific evidence to indicate that any of these are significantly effective at improving the incidence or severity of hot flushes. DHEA supplementation and isoflavones on the other hand have been shown, in a few small trials, to decrease the incidence of hot flushes and to improve measures of quality of life.

Mostly though this area has not been explored sufficiently and more rigorous investigations need to be done before it is clear which complementary medicines are effective in improving the symptoms of menopause and sleep during this time.

Behavioural therapies

Behavioural therapies aim to minimise the stress response. This is not to suggest that a woman in menopause is any more stressed than previously – it is just that during this stage of life her body, due to its decreasing level of oestrogen, cannot dampen even the most minor temperature response to the stress hormone noradrenaline. Some examples of behavioural therapies include:

- Yoga is a combination of exercise and meditation that involves gentle stretching and breath control. It has repeatedly been shown to decrease the severity and incidence of hot flushes and night sweats.

- Relaxation, including paced breathing, meditation and progressive relaxation. All have been shown to decrease the symptoms of menopause and improve the incidence and severity of hot flushes.
- Hypnosis has also been found to be useful in the management of hot flushes and night sweats, reducing the incidence of flushes by about 60%.
- CBT, which we have discussed in Chapter 7, is also showing some promising results. CBT promotes positive thoughts over negative thoughts and minimises the stress response.

Lifestyle modifications

There are some lifestyle modifications women going through menopause can make to help their sleeping as much as possible.

- Weight loss: avoiding weight gain as you age can be difficult but it is an important factor in your ability to maintain sleep during this period. Excess weight puts your body under considerable stress and predisposes you to chronic diseases such as type 2 diabetes, hypertension, heart disease and sleep apnoea, which in turn cause considerable sleep disturbance. Being overweight can also increase back pain and the level of pain felt generally, so that it is likely that you will experience multiple awakenings due to the greater discomfort and the need to change sleeping position to alleviate the stress on certain parts of the body. So if you have found the kilos creeping on, undertake some lifestyle changes that include a diet of healthy whole foods and 20–30 minutes of daily exercise.
- Limit hot and spicy foods and hot beverages and caffeine: when we drink or eat hot foods we can increase our body temperature. Due to the lack of the thermo-neutral zone in women experiencing hot flushes, any increase in temperature, no matter what the cause, can initiate the flush. So it is better to stick with cool drinks and non-spicy foods.
- Wear light, layered clothing: if you are wearing too much clothing, you will increase your body temperature (even by just a little bit) which can be sufficient to initiate a flush. So make

sure that you wear layered clothing that allows you to adapt to changing ambient temperatures.

- Cool the room at night: this is essential to reduce the effect of any night sweat you experience. As your body is susceptible to even the most minor change in temperature, keeping the room cool (17–18°C) will minimise the risk of getting warm and thereby initiating a flush. For those women who do not have airconditioning a fan works well and is also a good source of white noise (Chapter 15).
- Use breathable bedding and night wear: many mattresses, bed linen and nightwear are made of synthetic fibre which does not breathe well. If the heat generated by our (and any partner's) body cannot escape through our clothing or bedding we will start to warm up. For women of a certain age this is not a good thing. By having all bed clothing (linen as well as the bed itself) made of natural fibre you will minimise this happening. If you have just bought a new mattress not of natural material, overlay it with a cotton or wool cover – this will go some way to reducing the heating due to non-breathable materials.
- Good sleep practices: being diligent about your sleep habits is important at any time in life but especially now when sleep can become that little more elusive. Make sure you follow the top 10 tips outlined in Chapter 15.
- Exercise maintenance: exercise has been shown repeatedly to improve sleep. While this is one of the sleep tips already referred to above, it is so important that it has its own separate mention.

By implementing some of the interventions and strategies outlined above you should start to experience an improvement in your ability to sleep and begin again to have deep, restful sleep. If you find you still wake up occasionally with a night sweat, and find it difficult to get back to sleep, it is a good idea to start implementing the steps outlined in Chapter 9 (where we discussed sleep-maintenance insomnia) because even though the awakening from sleep is due to a specific reason, the why and how of getting back to sleep is still the same.

The stages of a woman's life – puberty, pregnancy and menopause – can be defining periods. They mark the end of one phase and the start of the next. These times should be welcomed and enjoyed and not dominated by overwhelming feelings of tiredness that make coping with the inherent changes more difficult. By recognising that these times can also be times of sleep difficulties and implementing the strategies suggested in this chapter it is possible to minimise the negative effects and enhance the many positive aspects of the new phase.

Sleep and mood diary

Over the next 2 months use the following table to rate how much you slept and how well you slept and felt each day of your cycle. Rate on a scale of 0 (when symptoms were non-existent) through to +++ (when symptoms were severe). If the symptoms are minimal in the first phase of the cycle (up until about day 14) but increase over the next 2 weeks and then start to reduce after the first few days of bleeding then it is likely that mood and sleep symptoms are a result of your hormonal cycle. If so, it is important to adopt the strategies outlined in this chapter.

Day of cycle	Last night I slept for:	Last night I had:			Today I felt:		
	# hours	Difficulty getting to sleep	Difficulty staying asleep	No difficulty sleeping	Unrefreshed when I awoke	Tired	Down
1							
2							
3							
4							
5							
6							
7							
8							
9							
10							
11							
12							
13							
14							
15							
16							
17							
18							
19							
20							
21							
22							
23							
24							
25							
26							
27							
28							
29							
30							
31							

Chapter 18

Sleeping aids

THROUGHOUT THIS BOOK I HAVE placed great emphasis on the importance of actively addressing our sleeping difficulties and of not relying on pharmacological sleeping aids. I believe strongly that this is the most beneficial and sustainable approach. That is not to say, however, that there is no place for sleeping aids.

On the contrary, sleep medications can play an important role in assisting people at particular times in their lives. It may be that, despite all that you have read in this book, you have come to a time in your life where you are absolutely desperate for sleep and have decided that the only workable solution in the short term is a sleep medication.

There are a few circumstances where taking a sleeping medication, provided it is used judiciously, may be a practical and workable consideration.

Jet lag

Sleeping aids can be especially useful when travelling across time zones and can assist in allowing sleep even when our circadian rhythms are not ready for sleep. For this reason many travellers will use them for the first few nights in a new destination. Care does need to be taken, however, as in these circumstances any drowsiness felt the next day may be worsened because of the sleep aid and as a result driving is strongly contraindicated.

Sleep aids taken to overcome the effects of jet lag need only be taken for the first 2–3 nights because after this time the body's circadian rhythms should have substantially adapted to the new time zone.

Emotional upheaval

Sleep aids may also give much-needed relief and allow sleep when we encounter some extreme emotional upset. This could be a relationship break-up, the death of a loved one, a very difficult time at work, or another circumstance. At these times sleep will be difficult and it is common for people to suffer sleeplessness.

As we know lack of sleep at any time can cause us to feel less positive about life, impair our thinking, decrease our motivation levels and make us susceptible to colds and flus. Clearly all these negative consequences will be acutely exacerbated during times of emotional or social upheavals and so any life event that seriously upsets us is only going to be made worse by a lack of sleep.

At times like these it may be an option to take a sleeping aid. Keep in mind, though, that sleeping aids should not be the first option and only taken if you really cannot sleep, despite following best sleep practice. If you decide to take a sleep medication it is advisable to follow these guidelines:

1. Rather than opting immediately for a prescription sleeping pill try a natural sleep aid first (discussed later in this chapter).
2. Take the medication for the shortest time possible; a few days may be sufficient to get you over the initial shock.
3. Do not take the sleeping aid for longer than a 2–4 week period.
4. If you do not need to take it every night – don't. Sometimes taking a sleeping aid just occasionally can get you over a difficult few nights.
5. Do not take the sleeping aid in combination with alcohol or illicit drugs.

6. Do not take sleeping aids while pregnant or breastfeeding unless under your doctor's advice.
7. While taking the sleeping aid it is crucial to be diligent about sleep practices, to exercise at least a little every day and to carry out a relaxation practice every evening. By doing this, at the end of the 2–4 week period you should have established a good sleep behaviour, which will give you the greatest chance of sleeping without the help of medication.
8. If, despite your best efforts, at the end of the 2–4 week period you are still unable to sleep well it is important that you consult your doctor to discuss your sleep difficulties. A counsellor may also be able to help you manage the emotional difficulties you are encountering.

Pain

Sometimes sleep is difficult due to physical pain. When we are in pain, we will find it hard to maintain sleep and our sleep will often be disturbed, which results in a state of sleep deprivation. It is an unfortunate fact that lack of sleep decreases our pain threshold so that we feel any pain more keenly.

In most situations pain should be managed by appropriate pain medication, but in circumstances where, despite adequate medication, there is continued sleeplessness a sleeping aid may help. In these circumstances a sleeping pill should only be taken in consultation with your doctor and only in the short-term, because even if the pain continues there is a fairly quick habituation to the sleeping aid. This means that if we choose to continue to take the medication we will need more of it to be effective, and if we do this we run the risk of building a reliance – either physically or psychologically – on the sleeping aid to get to, or maintain, sleep.

For this reason, managing sleep in circumstances of chronic pain is difficult and needs to be done under specialist care. In these cases, sleeping pills are often not the answer as they can only help in the short-term and chronic pain is an enduring state.

Choosing a sleeping aid

If, due to your current circumstances, you have decided that a sleeping aid is a real option the next question is what is the most suitable one for you? There is such a wide variety of sleeping aids available that deciding which one is best for your situation can be difficult. For the rest of this chapter we will look at some of the more commonly used sleep-enhancing medications, and the advantages and disadvantages of each.

Prescribed sleeping pills

Sleep medications available only by prescription from a medical practitioner are generally referred to as 'hypnotics'. All hypnotics work by depressing our central nervous system, which increases our sleepiness. Most of these drugs act on something known as the gamma-aminobutyric acid (GABA) receptor complex in our brain. GABA is a brain chemical (neurotransmitter) that sets in motion our brain's inhibitory pathways – in other words GABA is responsible for actively decreasing the levels of excitement and alertness in our brain and for promoting the feelings of calmness and quietness necessary for sleep. Anything that increases the effect of GABA will have a sleep-enhancing effect.

Currently, the most commonly prescribed groups of hypnotic drugs are benzodiazepines and other benzodiazepine-related drugs. They all work in the same way – they increase the activity of the GABA and deactivate the brain effectively 'knocking us out'. In Australia the most commonly prescribed sleeping pills are Valium, Mogadon, Xanax, Normison, Serepax, Stilnox and Imovane.

These drugs are categorised as short-, intermediate- or long-acting with the short- and intermediate-acting drugs being used mostly for the treatment of insomnia, and the longer-acting benzodiazepines for the treatment of anxiety. The table below summarises the type of effect and the half-life of these more common hypnotics. The complete list of prescribed hypnotics available in Australia is too long to be fully replicated in this table so if you do not recognise the sleeping pill you have been prescribed it would be worthwhile asking your doctor about it and about its half-life. It is important to know and understand the half-life of a drug as it is this that determines how long you will

Generic Name	Brand Name	Type of effect	Drug's duration of action (hours) (half-life)
	Benzodiazepines		
Nitrazepam	Mogadon, Alodorm	Long	16–48
Diazepam	Valium, Ducene, Antenex, Diazepam, Valpam	Long	> 20
Alprazolam	Xanax, Kalma, Alprax, Alprazolam, GENRX, Zamhexal	Intermediate	11–16
Oxazepam	Serepax, Murelax, Alepam	Intermediate	6–10
Temazepam	Normison, Temaze, Temtabs	Intermediate	8–20
	Benzodiazepine-related		
Zoplicone	Imovane, Imrest	Short	4.5–5.5
Zolpidem	Stilnox, Stilnoxium, Zolipdell, Dormizol, Somiden, Stildem	Short	1.5–2.4

be under the effects of the drug. The longer the half-life, the longer you will feel the sleep-enhancing actions of that medication.

As would be expected all the drugs listed in the above table have been proven to be effective at enhancing sleep and have been shown to:

- shorten the time it takes to fall asleep
- increase total sleep time
- decrease the number of awakenings
- improve sleep quality.

If you are experiencing jet lag, emotional or social upheaval or acute (short-term) pain and as a consequence are having a difficult time sleeping it may be that you need to take a hypnotic for a short time. It is important to realise, however, that although you will get these positive sleep outcomes you may also experience some less desirable consequences. While these drugs increase our total sleep time they do so by increasing the time we spend in stage 2 NREM sleep (our light sleep) and by decreasing both our deep sleep and REM sleep.

Given that these sleep stages are crucial to the restorative value of sleep for both our body and brain, it suggests that when we use these hypnotics we do not function optimally either physically or mentally. Certainly there are some clear and documented unwanted side effects and these include:

- excessive or daytime sedation (particularly with the intermediate-acting drugs)
- increased risk of falls (especially in the elderly) due to muscle relaxant effect
- decreased alertness and responsiveness the following morning (foggy-headedness) increasing the risk of accidents
- decreased cognitive ability the following morning
- amnesic effects, causing the person to forget events soon after taking a dose, including forgetting they took their medication
- disinhibited behaviour and hallucinations.

While these negative side effects are more likely to be experienced by those who use higher doses and/or hypnotics with longer half-lives, they can be experienced by anyone using sleeping pills.

A word of caution

Always remember that it is best to play it safe and that prescription sleeping pills are definitely not recommended and should not be taken if you:

- are pregnant or breastfeeding
- have, or think you have, sleep apnoea
- take illicit substances
- have advanced liver disease
- are a moderate–heavy user of alcohol

It would seem then that, to date, there is no perfect sleeping pill. There is, however, some good news – these days most of us are safe from building a physical dependence on sleeping pills as the ones used today are generally not physically addictive. That is not to say that people do not build up a strong psychological reliance on taking the sleeping pill to get to or maintain sleep, and this can be extremely difficult to overcome.

Therefore, whenever a decision is made, in consultation with your doctor, to take a prescription sleeping pill it is advisable firstly to trial a short-acting hypnotic at the lowest effective dose for the shortest possible period. It is also important that best sleep practices are implemented (Chapter 15) as these will give you the best chance of achieving deep and restful sleep on a regular basis without the need for any medication.

While there are circumstances where sleeping pills are appropriate and may provide much-needed sleep they should not be taken when another intervention may work as well – any underlying disorder needs to be recognised and treated, and sleep practices should be optimised before sleeping pills are used. It is also important to understand that sleep medication is a short-term solution only and that long-term continued use is not an option.

If though you find yourself in the situation of being a long-term user of sleeping pills and would like to stop, then switching to another type of sleeping pill is not the answer. It may be difficult to stop all of a sudden as this may cause rebound insomnia, which can be very perturbing. In this situation it is much more advisable to consult your doctor and together develop a strategy to reduce your reliance on sleeping pills.

Other prescription drugs

Antidepressants

There are several other drugs available by prescription which, while they do not work in the same way as the hypnotics discussed above, do have a sleep-enhancing effect and are sometimes used to treat insomnia. Most notable of these types of drugs are the tri-cyclic and tetra-cyclic antidepressants, such as Sinequan, Tryptanol, Surmontil, Avanza and Remeron, which may sometimes be prescribed at a sub-therapeutic dose because a sedative effect is one of the side effects. In general though, antidepressants should not be used to treat sleeplessness unless the person has also been diagnosed with depression. This is because tolerance to their sedative effects soon develops and they can have significant unwanted side effects including:

- weight gain
- dry mouth
- constipation
- decreased libido
- adverse cardiac effects
- low blood pressure (increased risk of falls)

Further, unless depression has been diagnosed, there is minimal scientific evidence to support the efficacy of using antidepressants in the treatment of insomnia.

Melatonin

We have already discussed at length the role of melatonin in the sleep process (Chapter 3). As we have learned, melatonin is secreted during the dark hours between sunset and sunrise and without sufficient melatonin we will find it difficult to get to, and/or maintain sleep.

There have been many placebo-controlled trials that have evaluated the efficacy of supplemental melatonin. The vast majority of these show that melatonin, when taken orally, has a sleep-enhancing effect, particularly in assisting sleep onset. For this reason it is particularly useful for jet lag and shift-work. The added advantage with using melatonin as a sleeping aid is that there appears to be no substantive negative side effects (the most commonly reported side effect being headache) and a minimal risk of physiological or psychological dependence.

Given its proven therapeutic effects it may be of value trialling melatonin as a first attempt to overcome sleeplessness. It is worthwhile noting that in many countries melatonin is an over-the-counter drug and is viewed as a herbal therapy, but in Australia, with the exception of homeopathic melatonin, it is only available with a doctor's prescription. The homeopathic preparations have been shown to have no effect on aiding sleep, because the amount of melatonin in these compounds is sub-therapeutic. Generally, the dose of melatonin required to obtain its sleep-enhancing effect varies with individuals from 3–6 mg. This is significantly greater than the amount of melatonin found in the homeopathic compounds. For this reason, if you decide that you would prefer to try melatonin instead of a sleeping pill you will need to consult your doctor.

Over-the-counter drugs

Antihistamines

Most over-the-counter products sold as night-time sleep aids contain an antihistamine, such as doxylamine or diphenydramine. While these are normally used to treat the symptoms of allergies people often use them to enhance sleep because they have sleepiness as a side effect. While they may be effective in the (very) short-term, they reduce the quality of sleep and a tolerance to them develops within days, meaning that a higher dose will be required for the medication to work. Moreover they can have prominent side effects including blurred vision, confusion and dizziness, especially in children and the elderly. They are therefore not recommended for overcoming sleeping difficulties.

Herbal therapies

For thousands of years plants have been used to aid sleep and today there are countless numbers of herbal preparations that are sold with the promise of improving sleep. Nearly all such herbal remedies will variously contain a combination of valerian *(Valeriana officinalis)*, hops *(Humulus lupulus)*, ginseng, passion flower *(Passiflora incarnata)* and kava kava *(Piper methysticum)*.

All commercially available herbal medications are regulated in terms of safety, however manufacturers of these medications are not required to provide data on their purity or their efficacy. For this reason it is difficult to determine exactly what preparations are effective in aiding sleep. This problem is further exacerbated by the fact that the active ingredients in a plant are determined by the particular species of the plant and where it is grown, so unless all trials of a particular herb are done with the same species and grown in the same area, results will be confounded – as indeed they are.

That is not to say that herbal medications do not work. Some are very effective, but these are usually ones that have undergone clinical testing and have results that back up their claims. If you are thinking about taking a herbal preparation it is critical to realise that not all of the preparations available on the market will be effective because the amount of the active ingredient has to be sufficient to evoke the desired sleep-enhancing effect. It is worthwhile doing a little bit of research and choosing only those preparations that have undergone clinical efficacy testing. Normally this information is easily obtained as most manufacturers of herbal remedies are keen to publicise when one of their preparations has had a positive outcome in a scientific clinical trial.

L-tryptophan

We have spoken briefly about L-tryptophan in Chapter 16 when we discussed its role as a building block for melatonin. L-tryptophan is an amino acid that is found in plants and animals and, in clinical trials, doses of 1 gm have been found to mildly improve the time it takes to get to sleep, as well as improving sleep maintenance. As it is found in the plants and animals we eat, however, if we maintain a healthy, whole food diet we should not require dietary supplementation. Despite this fact though many herbal sleep aids will contain this along with various combinations of the herbs discussed above. As mentioned there, it is important that we do a little research to determine that claims made by the manufacturer are verified by clinical studies, otherwise we could be wasting our money.

We could spend a considerably greater amount of time detailing the variety of sleep medications available today. What I have presented here is just a small overview of what we may be confronted with if we are considering taking a sleep medication, be it prescription, non-prescription or herbal. The available array is vast and can be confusing, especially so if we are already thinking more slowly due to sleep deprivation.

Whatever medication we eventually decide upon it is important to remember that it is not a permanent solution to our sleeplessness. If we find that after 2–4 weeks of use we are still relying on it to help us get to sleep, or to maintain sleep, then it is time to further investigate exactly what is causing our sleep difficulties. The best solution to overcoming poor sleep is to treat the cause and not the effect.

Chapter 19

The final step

BEFORE I GIVE THE FINAL step on achieving deep, restful sleep I thought I would share one more piece of research to encourage you to get the sleep you need – it appears that getting the right amount of sleep also makes us more attractive.

In a number of studies where participants have been deliberately sleep deprived, it has been found that after a night of little sleep people look rougher, with redder, more swollen eyes, darker under-eye circles, more wrinkles and droopier eyelids and mouths than their well-rested selves. People also looked sadder than after a normal sleep.

Taken all together it would appear then that the concept of a 'beauty sleep' is well based. This difference in appearance is borne out in a clinical trial that involved people with sleep apnoea. A photo was taken of twenty people who had been diagnosed with sleep apnoea, just before they commenced CPAP therapy. After 2 months of therapy, when the person's sleep apnoea had been treated and they had been having good, consolidated sleep for many weeks, another photo was taken. Independent assessors viewed the images side by side (the order of presentation of the 'pre' and 'post' photos varied) and rated them for alertness, youthfulness and attractiveness. In nearly all cases the assessors ranked the 'after' image more attractive and younger than the 'before' shot.

So, if renewed vitality and good health were not reason enough for us to focus on getting good sleep, there is now the added benefit of knowing that deep, restful sleep will make us look younger and more attractive.

We now have so many reasons to improve our sleep and if we follow the steps and strategies set out in this book we will be well on our way to achieving deep, restful sleep.

There is however, one final step – the need to monitor our sleep and track our improvements.

There are a number of sleep apps now available, some of which are good – so if this appeals to you find out which one you think might work for you. If you are more old school, or just like to keep a written diary, there is a morning and evening sleep diary provided in the appendix.

Whatever form of record you decide to keep, you need to monitor your sleep for at least 3 weeks. This timeframe is important because there is some research indicating that it takes at least 18 days to form or change a habit. So keeping a diary for less than 3 weeks means that it is more than likely that you will sink back into your old habits once your sleep starts to improve.

Noting the changes in your sleep, and tracking the nightly quality and quantity, will also allow you to assess your sleep practices and enable you to detect your own, individual sleep stealers (for example, drinking alcohol or having coffee too late in the day) and sleep enhancers (for example, turning off the computer early or exercising during the day). This will help you understand why some nights you do not sleep well and inform you as to what changes are needed in order for you to achieve good sleep.

Tracking your sleep also makes it possible for you to perceive when improvements begin to happen – even if they are only minor. This is important because it is easy to get discouraged if we don't see or feel almost immediate change. Keep in mind the wise Chinese saying: 'A journey of a thousand miles starts with a single step', and rejoice in each improvement that you see and feel.

Conclusion

I hope you have enjoyed reading this book as much as I have enjoyed writing it. I have been fascinated by the world of sleep for a long time now and have spent close on 20 years studying it. When I first started in this area very little was known about what happens to our body and brain during sleep, but this has all changed radically. Unfortunately, everything we know about sleep today has not filtered into our general knowledge yet and this is why I wrote this book.

Until recently, the best we could offer someone with sleeping difficulties was the 'good sleep tips' and sleeping medications. Good sleep practices play an important role in how well we are able to sleep, but they are only part of the solution. By taking the time to examine our specific sleep pattern and considering how this fits within the body's 24-hour rhythms; by working out whether we might have a sleep disorder; and by reflecting upon whether our daytime behaviours and stress levels are impacting on our sleep, we will be well on our way to solving our sleeplessness.

I hope you now have a much greater understanding of sleep and have discovered the answers to any questions that may have puzzled you about your sleep. Most importantly, I hope you now realise that sleep is highly personalised and that the solution to your sleep difficulties lies in understanding your own individual sleep needs and patterns. When we begin to understand the causes of *our* sleeplessness we can implement a process – or a set of steps as has been set out in this book – that will address the core problem. By getting at this core we can work both from the inside (our body and brain) and out (our behaviours) to solve the core problem and enable our sleep processes to flow easily and naturally.

As with any other lifestyle changes we decide to make, getting to the essential reason for your sleeplessness may take time and commitment, but once you have found the reason you can implement a cure. Realise that deep, restful sleep is just around the corner – and it is only you that can take you there.

Good luck!

Carmel

APPENDICES

Appendix 1

WEEK ONE
MORNING SLEEP DIARY – to be filled in every morning

	I went to bed last night at:	I got out of bed this morning at:	Last night I fell asleep in about:	I woke up during the night:	My sleep was disturbed by:	Last night I slept for a total of:	When I woke up for the day, I felt:
Morning of Day 1 Day ______ Date ______	______ am/pm	______ am/pm	______ minutes	______ times		______ hours	☐ Refreshed ☐ Somewhat refreshed ☐ Tired ☐ Very tired
Morning of Day 2 Day ______ Date ______	______ am/pm	______ am/pm	______ minutes	______ times		______ hours	☐ Refreshed ☐ Somewhat refreshed ☐ Tired ☐ Very tired
Morning of Day 3 Day ______ Date ______	______ am/pm	______ am/pm	______ minutes	______ times		______ hours	☐ Refreshed ☐ Somewhat refreshed ☐ Tired ☐ Very tired

Morning of Day 4 Day ________ Date ________	______ am/pm	______ am/pm	______ minutes	______ times		______ hours	☐ Refreshed ☐ Somewhat refreshed ☐ Tired ☐ Very tired
Morning of Day 5 Day ________ Date ________	______ am/pm	______ am/pm	______ minutes	______ times		______ hours	☐ Refreshed ☐ Somewhat refreshed ☐ Tired ☐ Very tired
Morning of Day 6 Day ________ Date ________	______ am/pm	______ am/pm	______ minutes	______ times		______ hours	☐ Refreshed ☐ Somewhat refreshed ☐ Tired ☐ Very tired
Morning of Day 7 Day ________ Date ________	______ am/pm	______ am/pm	______ minutes	______ times		______ hours	☐ Refreshed ☐ Somewhat refreshed ☐ Tired ☐ Very tired

Appendix 2

WEEK ONE EVENING SLEEP DIARY – to be filled in every evening						
	In the evening I ate (including dinner):	**I had caffeinated drinks during the:**	**I exercised at least 20 minutes in the:**	**Approximately 2–3 hours before going to bed, I had:**	**I napped during the:**	**1 hour before going to sleep, I did the following (*eg. smoked a cigarette, worked on the computer, watched TV, meditated, had a cup of tea etc.*):**
Evening of Day 1 Day ________ Date ________		Morning Afternoon 2–3 hours before bed I didn't have any	Morning Afternoon 2–3 hours before bed I didn't exercise	Alcohol A heavy meal A light snack Nothing	AM PM For: ________ minutes I didn't nap	
Evening of Day 2 Day ________ Date ________		Morning Afternoon 2–3 hours before bed I didn't have any	Morning Afternoon 2–3 hours before bed I didn't exercise	Alcohol A heavy meal A light snack Nothing	AM PM For: ________ minutes I didn't nap	
Evening of Day 3 Day ________ Date ________		Morning Afternoon 2–3 hours before bed I didn't have any	Morning Afternoon 2–3 hours before bed I didn't exercise	Alcohol A heavy meal A light snack Nothing	AM PM For: ________ minutes I didn't nap	

Evening of Day 4 Day ______ Date ______		Morning Afternoon 2–3 hours before bed I didn't have any	Morning Afternoon 2–3 hours before bed I didn't exercise	Alcohol A heavy meal A light snack Nothing	AM PM For: ______ minutes I didn't nap	
Evening of Day 5 Day ______ Date ______		Morning Afternoon 2–3 hours before bed I didn't have any	Morning Afternoon 2–3 hours before bed I didn't exercise	Alcohol A heavy meal A light snack Nothing	AM PM For: ______ minutes I didn't nap	
Evening of Day 6 Day ______ Date ______		Morning Afternoon 2–3 hours before bed I didn't have any	Morning Afternoon 2–3 hours before bed I didn't exercise	Alcohol A heavy meal A light snack Nothing	AM PM For: ______ minutes I didn't nap	
Evening of Day 7 Day ______ Date ______		Morning Afternoon 2–3 hours before bed I didn't have any	Morning Afternoon 2–3 hours before bed I didn't exercise	Alcohol A heavy meal A light snack Nothing	AM PM For: ______ minutes I didn't nap	

Appendix 3

WEEK TWO MORNING SLEEP DIARY – to be filled in every morning							
	I went to bed last night at:	I got out of bed this morning at:	Last night I fell asleep in about:	I woke up during the night:	My sleep was disturbed by:	Last night I slept for a total of:	When I woke up for the day, I felt:
Morning of Day 1 Day ______ Date ______	______ am/pm	______ am/pm	______ minutes	______ times		______ hours	☐ Refreshed ☐ Somewhat refreshed ☐ Tired ☐ Very tired
Morning of Day 2 Day ______ Date ______	______ am/pm	______ am/pm	______ minutes	______ times		______ hours	☐ Refreshed ☐ Somewhat refreshed ☐ Tired ☐ Very tired
Morning of Day 3 Day ______ Date ______	______ am/pm	______ am/pm	______ minutes	______ times		______ hours	☐ Refreshed ☐ Somewhat refreshed ☐ Tired ☐ Very tired

Morning of Day 4 Day ________ Date ________	______ am/pm	______ am/pm	______ minutes	______ times		______ hours	☐ Refreshed ☐ Somewhat refreshed ☐ Tired ☐ Very tired
Morning of Day 5 Day ________ Date ________	______ am/pm	______ am/pm	______ minutes	______ times		______ hours	☐ Refreshed ☐ Somewhat refreshed ☐ Tired ☐ Very tired
Morning of Day 6 Day ________ Date ________	______ am/pm	______ am/pm	______ minutes	______ times		______ hours	☐ Refreshed ☐ Somewhat refreshed ☐ Tired ☐ Very tired
Morning of Day 7 Day ________ Date ________	______ am/pm	______ am/pm	______ minutes	______ times		______ hours	☐ Refreshed ☐ Somewhat refreshed ☐ Tired ☐ Very tired

Appendix 4

WEEK TWO EVENING SLEEP DIARY – to be filled in every evening						
	In the evening I ate (including dinner):	I had caffeinated drinks during the:	I exercised at least 20 minutes in the:	Approximately 2–3 hours before going to bed, I had:	I napped during the:	1 hour before going to sleep, I did the following (*eg. smoked a cigarette, worked on the computer, watched TV, meditated, had a cup of tea etc.*):
Evening of Day 8 Day ________ Date ________		Morning Afternoon 2–3 hours before bed I didn't have any	Morning Afternoon 2–3 hours before bed I didn't exercise	Alcohol A heavy meal A light snack Nothing	AM PM For: ______ minutes I didn't nap	
Evening of Day 9 Day ________ Date ________		Morning Afternoon 2–3 hours before bed I didn't have any	Morning Afternoon 2–3 hours before bed I didn't exercise	Alcohol A heavy meal A light snack Nothing	AM PM For: ______ minutes I didn't nap	
Evening of Day 10 Day ________ Date ________		Morning Afternoon 2–3 hours before bed I didn't have any	Morning Afternoon 2–3 hours before bed I didn't exercise	Alcohol A heavy meal A light snack Nothing	AM PM For: ______ minutes I didn't nap	

Evening of Day 11 Day ________ Date ________		Morning Afternoon 2–3 hours before bed I didn't have any	Morning Afternoon 2–3 hours before bed I didn't exercise	Alcohol A heavy meal A light snack Nothing	AM PM For: _______ minutes I didn't nap	
Evening of Day 12 Day ________ Date ________		Morning Afternoon 2–3 hours before bed I didn't have any	Morning Afternoon 2–3 hours before bed I didn't exercise	Alcohol A heavy meal A light snack Nothing	AM PM For: _______ minutes I didn't nap	
Evening of Day 13 Day ________ Date ________		Morning Afternoon 2–3 hours before bed I didn't have any	Morning Afternoon 2–3 hours before bed I didn't exercise	Alcohol A heavy meal A light snack Nothing	AM PM For: _______ minutes I didn't nap	
Evening of Day 14 Day ________ Date ________		Morning Afternoon 2–3 hours before bed I didn't have any	Morning Afternoon 2–3 hours before bed I didn't exercise	Alcohol A heavy meal A light snack Nothing	AM PM For: _______ minutes I didn't nap	

Appendix 5

WEEK THREE
MORNING SLEEP DIARY – to be filled in every morning

	I went to bed last night at:	I got out of bed this morning at:	Last night I fell asleep in about:	I woke up during the night:	My sleep was disturbed by:	Last night I slept for a total of:	When I woke up for the day, I felt:
Morning of Day 15 Day ________ Date ________	________ am/pm	________ am/pm	________ minutes	________ times		________ hours	☐ Refreshed ☐ Somewhat refreshed ☐ Tired ☐ Very tired
Morning of Day 16 Day ________ Date ________	________ am/pm	________ am/pm	________ minutes	________ times		________ hours	☐ Refreshed ☐ Somewhat refreshed ☐ Tired ☐ Very tired
Morning of Day 17 Day ________ Date ________	________ am/pm	________ am/pm	________ minutes	________ times		________ hours	☐ Refreshed ☐ Somewhat refreshed ☐ Tired ☐ Very tired

Morning of Day 18 Day ______ Date ______	______ am/pm	______ am/pm	______ minutes	______ times		______ hours	☐ Refreshed ☐ Somewhat refreshed ☐ Tired ☐ Very tired
Morning of Day 19 Day ______ Date ______	______ am/pm	______ am/pm	______ minutes	______ times		______ hours	☐ Refreshed ☐ Somewhat refreshed ☐ Tired ☐ Very tired
Morning of Day 20 Day ______ Date ______	______ am/pm	______ am/pm	______ minutes	______ times		______ hours	☐ Refreshed ☐ Somewhat refreshed ☐ Tired ☐ Very tired
Morning of Day 21 Day ______ Date ______	______ am/pm	______ am/pm	______ minutes	______ times		______ hours	☐ Refreshed ☐ Somewhat refreshed ☐ Tired ☐ Very tired

Appendix 6

WEEK THREE
EVENING SLEEP DIARY – to be filled in every morning

	In the evening I ate (including dinner):	**I had caffeinated drinks during the:**	**I exercised at least 20 minutes in the:**	**Approximately 2–3 hours before going to bed, I had:**	**I napped during the:**	**1 hour before going to sleep, I did the following (*eg. smoked a cigarette, worked on the computer, watched TV, meditated, had a cup of tea etc.*):**
Evening of Day 15 Day ________ Date ________		Morning Afternoon 2–3 hours before bed I didn't have any	Morning Afternoon 2–3 hours before bed I didn't exercise	Alcohol A heavy meal A light snack Nothing	AM PM For: ________ minutes I didn't nap	
Evening of Day 16 Day ________ Date ________		Morning Afternoon 2–3 hours before bed I didn't have any	Morning Afternoon 2–3 hours before bed I didn't exercise	Alcohol A heavy meal A light snack Nothing	AM PM For: ________ minutes I didn't nap	
Evening of Day 17 Day ________ Date ________		Morning Afternoon 2–3 hours before bed I didn't have any	Morning Afternoon 2–3 hours before bed I didn't exercise	Alcohol A heavy meal A light snack Nothing	AM PM For: ________ minutes I didn't nap	

Evening of Day 18 Day ________ Date ________		Morning Afternoon 2–3 hours before bed I didn't have any	Morning Afternoon 2–3 hours before bed I didn't exercise	Alcohol A heavy meal A light snack Nothing	AM PM For: ________ minutes I didn't nap	
Evening of Day 19 Day ________ Date ________		Morning Afternoon 2–3 hours before bed I didn't have any	Morning Afternoon 2–3 hours before bed I didn't exercise	Alcohol A heavy meal A light snack Nothing	AM PM For: ________ minutes I didn't nap	
Evening of Day 20 Day ________ Date ________		Morning Afternoon 2–3 hours before bed I didn't have any	Morning Afternoon 2–3 hours before bed I didn't exercise	Alcohol A heavy meal A light snack Nothing	AM PM For: ________ minutes I didn't nap	
Evening of Day 21 Day ________ Date ________		Morning Afternoon 2–3 hours before bed I didn't have any	Morning Afternoon 2–3 hours before bed I didn't exercise	Alcohol A heavy meal A light snack Nothing	AM PM For: ________ minutes I didn't nap	

References

Introduction

Buysse, D. J. (2013). 'Insomnia', *Journal of the American Medical Association*, 309(7): 706–716.

Chapter 1

Cappuccio, F. P., D. Cooper, et al. (2011). 'Sleep duration predicts cardiovascular outcomes: a systematic review and meta-analysis of prospective studies', *European Heart Journal*, 32(12): 1484–1492.

Cappuccio, F. P., L. D'Elia, et al. (2010). 'Sleep duration and all-cause mortality: a systematic review and meta-analysis of prospective studies', *Sleep*, 33(5): 585–592.

Gomes, A. A., J. Tavares, et al. (2011). 'Sleep and academic performance in undergraduates: a multi-measure, multi-predictor approach', *Chronobiology International*, 28(9): 786–801.

Grandner, M. A. and M. L. Perlis (2013). 'Insomnia as a cardiometabolic risk factor', *Sleep*, 36(1): 11–12.

Grandner, M. A., M. R. Sands-Lincoln, et al. (2013). 'Sleep duration, cardiovascular disease, and proinflammatory biomarkers', *Nature and Science of Sleep*, 5: 93–107.

Kripke, D. F., R. D. Langer, et al. (2012). 'Hypnotics' association with mortality or cancer: a matched cohort study', *BMJ Open*, 2(1): e000850 doi: 10.1136/bmjopen-2012–000850

Mitler, M. M., M. A. Carskadon, et al. (1988). 'Catastrophes, sleep, and public policy: consensus report', *Sleep*, 11(1): 100–109.

Osorio, R. S., E. Pirraglia, et al. (2011). 'Greater risk of Alzheimer's disease in older adults with insomnia', *Journal of the American Geriatric Society*, 59(3): 559–562.

Van Dongen, H. P., G. Maislin, et al. (2003). 'The cumulative cost of additional wakefulness: dose-response effects on neurobehavioral functions and sleep physiology from chronic sleep restriction and total sleep deprivation', *Sleep*, 26(2): 117–126.

Chapter 2

Carskadon, M. A. and W. C. Dement (2011). 'Normal Human Sleep', *Principles and Practices of Sleep Medicine*, Kryger, M. H., T. Roth and W. C. Dement, Elsevier Saunders, St. Louis, Missouri, pages 470–482.

He, Y., C. R. Jones, et al. (2009). 'The transcriptional repressor DEC2 regulates sleep length in mammals', *Science*, 325(5942): 866–870.

Millstein, J., C. J. Winrow, et al. (2011). 'Identification of causal genes, networks, and transcriptional regulators of REM sleep and wake', *Sleep*, 34(11): 1469–1477

Chapter 3

Dement, W. C. and C. Vaughan (1999). *The Promise of Sleep*, Dell Publishing, New York, pages 102–124.

Seidel, W. F., S. Ball, et al. (1984). 'Daytime alertness in relation to mood, performance, and nocturnal sleep in chronic insomniacs and noncomplaining sleepers', *Sleep*, 7(3): 230–238.

Chapter 4

Arroll, B., A. Fernando III, et al. (2012). 'Prevalence of causes of insomnia in primary care: a cross-sectional study', *British Journal of General Practice*, 62(595): e99–103.

Bastien, C. H., Vallieres, A., Morin, C. M. (2001). 'Validation of the Insomnia Severity Index as an outcome measure for insomnia research', *Sleep Medicine*, 2(4): 297–307.

Chapter 5

Arroll, B., A. Fernando III, et al. (2012). 'Prevalence of causes of insomnia in primary care: a cross-sectional study', *British Journal of General Practice*, 62(595): e99–103.

Spitzer, R. L., K. Kroenke, et al. (2006). 'A brief measure for assessing generalized anxiety disorder: the GAD-7', *Archives of Internal Medicine*, 166(10): 1092–1097.

Chapter 6

Beck, A.T. (2005). *Anxiety Disorders and Phobias: A cognitive perspective*, Basic Books, New York.

Grandner, M. A., D. F. Kripke, et al. (2010). 'Relationships among dietary nutrients and subjective sleep, objective sleep, and napping in women', *Sleep Medicine*, 11(2): 180–184.

Khoury, B., T. Lecomte, et al. (2013). 'Mindfulness-based therapy: a comprehensive meta analysis', *Clinical Psychology Review*, 33(6): 763–771.

Youngstedt, S. D. (2005). 'Effects of exercise on sleep', *Clinical Sports Medicine*, 24(2): 355–365.

Chapter 7

Buysse, D. J., A. Germain, et al. (2011). 'Efficacy of brief behavioral treatment for chronic insomnia in older adults', *Archives of Internal Medicine*, 171(10): 887–895.

Vincent, N. and S. Lewycky (2009). 'Logging on for better sleep: RCT of the effectiveness of online treatment for insomnia', *Sleep*, 32(6): 807–815.

Chapter 8

Youngstedt, S. D. (2005). 'Effects of exercise on sleep', *Clinical Sports Medicine*, 24(2): 355–365.

Chapter 9

Dement, W. C. and C. Vaughan (1999). *The Promise of Sleep*, Dell Publishing, New York, pages 102–124.

Ekirch, A. R. (2005). *At Day's Close: Night in Times Past*, The Orion Publishing Group, United Kingdom, pages 301–303.

Taylor, D. J., K. L. Lichstein, et al. (2005). 'Epidemiology of insomnia, depression, and anxiety', *Sleep*, 28(11): 1457–1464.

Chapter 10

Edinger, J. D. and A. D. Krystal (2003). 'Subtyping primary insomnia: Is sleep state misperception a distinct clinical entity?', *Sleep Medicine Review*, 7(3): 203–214.

Chapter 11

American Academy of Sleep Medicine (2005). *International Classification of Sleep Disorders*, second edition, American Academy of Sleep Medicine, Darien, Illinois.

Arroll, B., A. Fernando III, et al. (2012). 'Prevalence of causes of insomnia in primary care: a cross-sectional study', *British Journal of General Practice*, 62(595): e99–103.

Kryger, M. H., T. Roth and W. C. Dement (2011). *Principles and Practices of Sleep Medicine*, Elsevier Saunders, St. Louis, Missouri.

Patrick, L. R. (2007). 'Restless legs syndrome: pathophysiology and the role of iron and folate', *Alternative Medicine Review*, 12(2): 101–112.

Reid, K. J. and P. C. Zee (2011). 'Circadian disorders of the sleep-wake cycle', *Principles and Practices of Sleep Medicine*, Kryger, M. H., T. Roth and W.C. Dement, Elsevier Saunders, St. Louis, Missouri, pages 470–482.

Chapter 12

Arroll, B., A. Fernando III, et al. (2012). 'Prevalence of causes of insomnia in primary care: a cross-sectional study', *British Journal of General Practice*, 62(595): e99–103.

Budweiser, S., R. Luigart, et al. (2013). 'Long-term changes of sexual function in men with obstructive sleep apnea after initiation of continuous positive airway pressure', *Journal of Sexual Medicine*, 10(2): 524–531.

Lurie, A. (2011). 'Obstructive sleep apnea in adults: epidemiology, clinical presentation, and treatment options', *Advanced Cardiology*, 46: 1–42.

Petersen, M., E. Kristensen, et al. (2011). 'Sexual function in female patients with obstructive sleep apnea', *Journal of Sexual Medicine*, 8(9): 2560–2568.

Vijayan, V. K. (2012). 'Morbidities associated with obstructive sleep apnea', *Expert Reviews in Respiratory Medicine*, 6(5): 557–566.

Young, T., M. Palta, et al. (2009). 'Burden of sleep apnea: rationale, design, and major findings of the Wisconsin Sleep Cohort study', *Wisconsin Medical Journal*, 108(5): 246–249.

Young, T., L. Finn, et al. (2008). 'Sleep disordered breathing and mortality: eighteen year follow-up of the Wisconsin sleep cohort', *Sleep*, 31(8): 1071–1078.

Chapter 13

Bolla, K. I., S. R. Lesage, et al. (2010). 'Polysomnogram changes in marijuana users who report sleep disturbances during prior abstinence', *Sleep Medicine*, 11(9): 882–89.

Rickwood, D., L. Magor-Blatch, et al. (2008). 'Substance use. A position statement prepared for the Australian Psychological Society', Australian Psychological Society, Melbourne, Australia.

Roehrs, T. and T. Roth (2011). 'Medication and substance abuse', *Principles and Practices of Sleep Medicine*, Kryger, M. H., T. Roth and W. C. Dement, Elsevier Saunders, St. Louis, Missouri, pages 1512–1523.

Ross, J. (Ed) (2007). *Illicit Drug Use in Australia: Epidemiology, Use Patterns and Associated Harm*, second edition, National Drug and Alcohol Research Centre, Paper-based publications, Commonwealth of Australia.

Chapter 14

Arroll, B., A. Fernando III, et al. (2012). 'Prevalence of causes of insomnia in primary care: a cross-sectional study', *British Journal of General Practice*, 62(595): e99–103.

Buysse, D. J., A. Germain, et al. (2011). 'Efficacy of brief behavioral treatment for chronic insomnia in older adults', *Archives of Internal Medicine*, 171(10): 887–895.

Galuszko-Wegielnik, M., K. Jakuszkowiak-Wojten, et al. (2012). 'The efficacy of Cognitive-Behavioural Therapy (CBT) as related to sleep quality and hyperarousal level in the treatment of primary insomnia', *Psychiatrica Danubina*, 24 Suppl. 1: S51–55.

Morin, C. M., S. Rodrigue, et al. (2003). 'Role of stress, arousal, and coping skills in primary insomnia', *Psychosomatic Medicine*, 65(2): 259–267.

Petersen, M., E. Kristensen, et al. (2011). 'Sexual function in female patients with obstructive sleep apnea', *Journal of Sexual Medicine*, 8(9): 2560–2568.

Chapter 15

Bartlett, D. J., N. S. Marshall, et al. (2008). 'Sleep health New South Wales: chronic sleep restriction and daytime sleepiness', *Internal Medicine Journal*, 38(1): 24–31.

Basner, M., U. Muller, et al. (2011). 'Single and combined effects of air, road, and rail traffic noise on sleep and recuperation', *Sleep*, 34(1): 11–23.

Buxton, O. M., C. W. Lee, et al. (2003). 'Exercise elicits phase shifts and acute alterations of melatonin that vary with circadian phase', *American Journal of Physiology: Regulatory, integrative and comparative physiology*, 284(3): R714–724.

Crispim, C. A., I. Z. Zimberg, et al. (2011). 'Relationship between food intake and sleep pattern in healthy individuals', *Journal of Clinical Sleep Medicine*, 7(6): 659–664.

Jaehne, A., B. Loessl, et al. (2009). 'Effects of nicotine on sleep during consumption, withdrawal and replacement therapy', *Sleep Medicine Review*, 13(5): 363–377.

Kryger, M. H., T. Roth and W. C. Dement (2011). *Principles and Practices of Sleep Medicine*, Elsevier Saunders, St. Louis, Missouri.

National Sleep Foundation (2010). *Sleep in America Poll Summary of Findings*: http://www.sleepfoundation.org/sites/default/files/nsaw/NSF%20Sleep%20in%20%20America%20Poll%20-%20Summary%20of%20Findings%20.pdf

Omlin, S., G. F. Bauer, et al. (2011). 'Effects of noise from non-traffic-related ambient sources on sleep: review of the literature of 1990–2010', *Noise Health*, 13(53): 299–309.

Zhang, L., J. Samet, et al. (2008). 'Power spectral analysis of EEG activity during sleep in cigarette smokers', *Chest*, 133(2): 427–432.

Chapter 16

Choi, S., B. Disilvio, et al. (2009). 'Meal ingestion, amino acids and brain neurotransmitters: effects of dietary protein source on serotonin and catecholamine synthesis rates', *Physiology and Behaviour*, 98(1–2): 156–162.

Cohen, S., W. J. Doyle, et al. (2009). 'Sleep habits and susceptibility to the common cold', *Archives of Internal Medicine*, 169(1): 62–67.

Grandner, M. A., N. Jackson, et al. (2013). 'Dietary nutrients associated with short and long sleep duration. Data from a nationally representative sample.', *Appetite*, 64: 71–80.

——(2013). 'Sleep symptoms associated with intake of specific dietary nutrients', *Journal of Sleep Research*, doi: 10.1111/jsr.12084

Grandner, M. A., D. F. Kripke, et al. (2010). 'Relationships among dietary nutrients and subjective sleep, objective sleep, and napping in women', *Sleep Medicine*, 11(2): 180–84.

Hajak, G., G. Huether, et al. (1991). 'The influence of intravenous L-tryptophan on plasma melatonin and sleep in men', *Pharmacopsychiatry*, 24(1): 17–20.

Hartmann, E., J. Cravens, et al. (1974). 'Hypnotic effects of L-tryptophan', *Archives of General Psychiatry*, 31(3): 394–397.

Head, K. A. and G. S. Kelly (2009). 'Nutrients and botanicals for treatment of stress: adrenal fatigue, neurotransmitter imbalance, anxiety, and restless sleep', *Alternative Medicine Review*, 14(2): 114–140.

Irwin, M., J. McClintick, et al. (1996). 'Partial night sleep deprivation reduces natural killer and cellular immune responses in humans', *FASEB Journal*, 10(5): 643–653.

Lee, J., D. Kim, et al. (2004). 'Lack of delta waves and sleep disturbances during non-rapid eye movement sleep in mice lacking alpha1 G-subunit of T-type calcium channels', *Proceedings of the National Academy of Science USA*, 101(52): 18195–18199.

Markus, C. R., L. M. Jonkman, et al. (2005). 'Evening intake of alpha-lactalbumin increases plasma tryptophan availability and improves morning alertness and brain measures of attention', *American Journal of Clinical Nutrition*, 81(5): 1026–1033.

Nindl, B. C., W. C. Hymer, et al. (2001). 'Growth hormone pulsatility profile characteristics following acute heavy resistance exercise', *Journal of Applied Physiology*, 91(1): 163–72.

Pan, R. M., C. Mauron, et al. (1982). 'Effect of various oral glucose doses on plasma neutral amino acid levels,' *Metabolism*, 31(9): 937–943.

Rethorst, C. D., P. Sunderajan, et al. (2013). 'Does exercise improve self-reported sleep quality in non-remitted major depressive disorder?', *Psychological Medicine*, 43(4): 699–709.

Rondanelli, M., A. Opizzi, et al. (2011). 'The effect of melatonin, magnesium, and zinc on primary insomnia in long-term care facility residents in Italy: a double-blind, placebo-controlled clinical trial', *Journal of the American Geriatric Society*, 59(1): 82–90.

Thomas, G. A., W. J. Kraemer, et al. (2013). 'Obesity, growth hormone and exercise', *Sports Medicine*, 43(9): 839–849.

Wilder-Smith, A., F. B. Mustafa, et al. (2013). 'Impact of partial sleep deprivation on immune markers', *Sleep Medicine*, 14(10): 1031–1034.

Youngstedt, S. D. (2005). 'Effects of exercise on sleep', *Clinical Sports Medicine*, 24(2): 355–365, xi.

Chapter 17

Aidelsburger, P., S. Schauer, et al. (2012). 'Alternative methods for the treatment of post-menopausal troubles', *GMS Health Technology Assessment*, doi: 10.3205/hta000101

Archer, D. F., D. W. Sturdee, et al. (2011). 'Menopausal hot flushes and night sweats: where are we now?', *Climacteric*, 14(5): 515–528.

Baker, F. C., L. O'Brien, et al. (2011). 'Sex differences and menstrual related changes in sleep and circadian rhythms', *Principles and Practices of Sleep Medicine*, Kryger, M. H., T. Roth, and W. C. Dement, Elsevier Saunders, St. Louis, Missouri, pages 1562–1571.

Balserak, I. B., K. Lee (2011). 'Sleep disturbances and sleep related disorders in pregnancy', *Principles and Practices of Sleep Medicine*, Kryger, M. H., T. Roth, and W. C. Dement, Elsevier Saunders, St. Louis, Missouri, pages 1572–1586.

Bourjeily, G., G. Ankner, et al. (2011). 'Sleep-disordered breathing in pregnancy', *Clinics in Chest Medicine*, 32(1): 175–189, x.

Bourjeily, G., C. A. Raker, et al. (2010). 'Pregnancy and fetal outcomes of symptoms of sleep-disordered breathing', *European Respiratory Journal*, 36(4): 849–55.

Champagne, K. A., R. J. Kimoff, et al. (2010). 'Sleep disordered breathing in women of childbearing age and during pregnancy', *Indian Journal of Medical Research*, 131: 285–301.

Cook, F., J. Bayer, et al. (2012). 'Baby Business: a randomised controlled trial of a universal parenting program that aims to prevent early infant sleep and cry problems and associated parental depression', *BMC Pediatrics*, 12: 13.

Crawford, S. L., E. A. Jackson, et al. (2013). 'Impact of dose, frequency of administration,and equol production on efficacy of isoflavones for menopausal hot flashes: a pilot randomized trial', *Menopause*, 20(9): 911–921.

Darnall, B. D. and E. C. Suarez (2009). 'Sex and gender in psychoneuroimmunology research: past, present and future', *Brain Behavior and Immunity*, 23(5): 595–604.

Dormire, S. L. and R. Bongiovanni (2008). 'Norepinephrine activity, as measured by MHPG, is associated with menopausal hot flushes', *Climacteric*, 11(5): 397–403.

Freedman, R. R. (2001). 'Physiology of hot flashes', *American Journal of Human Biology*, 13(4): 453–464.

Hutchison, B. L., P. R. Stone, et al. (2012). 'A postal survey of maternal sleep in late pregnancy', *BMC Pregnancy Childbirth*, 12: 144.

Kravitz, H. M. and H. Joffe (2011). 'Sleep during the perimenopause: a SWAN story', *Obstetrics and Gynecology Clinics of North America*, 38(3): 567–86.

Lee, K. A., K. E. Moe (2011). 'Menopause', *Principles and Practices of Sleep Medicine*, Kryger, M. H., T. Roth and W. C., Dement, Elsevier Saunders, St. Louis, Missouri, pages 1592–1601.

Montgomery-Downs, H. E., S. P. Insana, et al. (2010). 'Normative longitudinal maternal sleep: the first 4 months', *American Journal of Obstetrics and Gynecology*, 203(5): 465, e461–67.

Morrow, P. K., D. N. Mattair, et al. (2011). 'Hot flashes: a review of pathophysiology and treatment modalities', *Oncologist*, 16(11): 1658–1664.

O'Brien, L. M., A. S. Bullough, et al. (2012). 'Pregnancy-onset habitual snoring, gestational hypertension, and preeclampsia: prospective cohort study', *American Journal of Obstetrics and Gynecology*, 207(6): 487, e481–489.

——(2013). 'Snoring during pregnancy and delivery outcomes: A cohort study', *Sleep*, 36(11): 1625–1632.

O'Brien, L. M., J. T. Owusu, et al. (2013). 'Habitual snoring and depressive symptoms during pregnancy', *BMC Pregnancy Childbirth*, 13(1): 113.

Pachman, D. R., J. M. Jones, et al. (2010). 'Management of menopause-associated vasomotor symptoms: Current treatment options, challenges and future directions', *International Journal of Women's Health*, 2: 123–135.

Quincy, B. (2013). 'Perimenopausal sleep disturbance: beyond estrogen replacement', *Journal of the American Academy of Physician Assistants*, 26(1): 50–54.

Schindler, A. E. (2013). 'Non-contraceptive benefits of oral hormonal contraceptives', *International Journal of Endocrinology and Metabolism*, 11(1): 41–47.

Shechter, A., P. Lesperance, et al. (2012). 'Nocturnal polysomnographic sleep across the menstrual cycle in premenstrual dysphoric disorder', *Sleep Medicine*, 13(8): 1071–1078.

Stremler, R. and A. R. Wolfson (2011). 'The post-partum period', *Principles and Practices of Sleep Medicine*, Kryger, M. H., T. Roth, and W. C. Dement, Elsevier Saunders, St. Louis, Missouri, pages 1587–1591.

Chapter 18

Gillin, J. C., T. Roehrs et al. (2013). 'Sleep aids and insomnia', National Sleep Foundation, http://www.sleepfoundation.org

Gooneratne, N. S., A. Tavaria, et al. (2011). 'Perceived effectiveness of diverse sleep treatments in older adults', *Journal of the American Geriatric Society*, 59(2): 297–303.

John, W. G. (2003). 'The management of insomnia: an update', *Australian Prescriber*, 26: 78–81.

Olson, L. G. (2008). 'Hypnotic hazards: adverse effects of zolipidem and other z-drugs', *Australian Prescriber*, 31: 146–149.

Proctor, A. and M. T. Bianchi (2012). 'Clinical pharmacology in sleep medicine', *ISRN Pharmacology*, doi: 10.5402/2012/914168

Robinson, L., G. Kemp (2013). 'Sleeping pills and natural sleep aids', http://www.helpguide.org

Chapter 19

Axelsson, J., T. Sundelin, et al. (2010). 'Beauty sleep: experimental study on the perceived health and attractiveness of sleep deprived people', *British Medical Journal*, 341: c6614.

Chervin, R. D., D. L. Ruzicka, et al. (2013). 'The face of sleepiness: improvement in appearance after treatment of sleep apnea', *Journal of Clinical Sleep Medicine*, 9(9): 845–852.

Graybiel, A. M. (2008). 'Habits, rituals, and the evaluative brain', *Annual Review of Neuroscience*, 31: 359–387.

Lally, P., C. H. M. van Jaarsveld, et al. (2010). 'How are habits formed: Modelling habit formation in the real world', *European Journal of Social Psychology*, 40: 998–1009.

Acknowledgements

MY THANKS AND APPRECIATION GO to the countless number of sleep researchers who have unravelled many of the mysteries of sleep – it is because of their work and dedication that this book could be written.

My special thanks also to the team that enabled my initial manuscript to become the book it is today – my agent Sophie Hamley, my publisher Ingrid Ohlsson and my editors Deonie Fiford and Vanessa Pellatt. Their encouragement and hard work made the process easy and enjoyable.

My appreciation and thanks to Jean Ellis, Susan Sortor-Leger and Leonie O'Sullivan whose continued support and belief in the work I do greatly facilitated my ability to complete this project.

To my children Alexander and Charlotte – thank you for always being so delightfully encouraging, regardless of the challenge I undertake. And finally, to my mainstay – my wonderful husband Steven. My heartfelt thanks for your love, optimism and constant enthusiasm.

Index

Jean Kittson

YOU'RE STILL HOT TO ME

A fact-filled conversation starter on menopause by comedian and health campaigner Jean Kittson.

When Jean Kittson hit menopause, she couldn't understand why it wasn't a topic for conversation among women. Seeing that 1.5 million Australian women are menopausal at any given time, and in a world where everything from drug addiction to Brazilian waxes is discussed, why, she wondered, was menopause still considered taboo?

Jean decided to discover the facts that would help break menopause out of the closet, throw it in a fabulous dress and march it through town. She interviewed many of Australia's top medical experts in the area, and dozens of women – friends, colleagues, hairdressers – who were experts on getting through menopause without causing (much) harm to others.

Jean gives us the lowdown on common symptoms (would you like hot flushes with that?), getting the medical attention we deserve, treatments that work (as opposed to those that merely drain our bank accounts), and how to still be talking to loved ones when we emerge.

Candid and frequently hilarious, this is your complete guide on how to make the most of, and even occasionally celebrate, this momentous time of life.

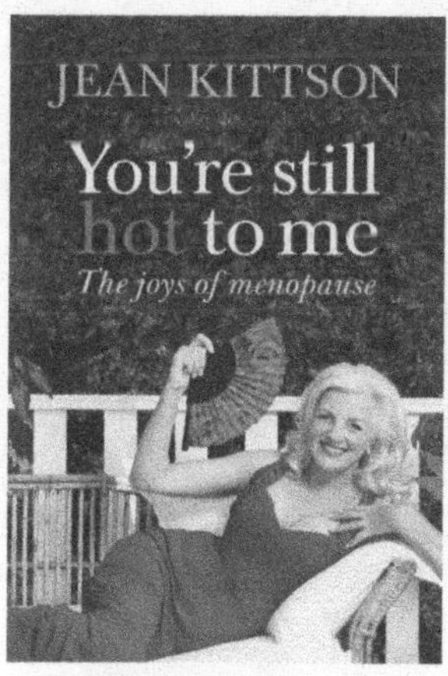

Dr Catherine Itsiopoulos (PhD APD)

THE MEDITERRANEAN DIET

This beautifully photographed book is your complete guide to the world's most famous, effective and sustainable diet by one of Australia's leading researchers.

The Mediterranean Diet is the diet on which others are based. Its positive health effects have been rigorously tested for more than 60 years, and the results are clear. The diet has been proven to prevent heart disease and diabetes, help with weight management, slow the progress of Alzheimer's and promote longevity.

Dr Catherine Itsiopoulos has spent her working life researching the diet. Drawing on the food traditions of her Greek heritage, Dr Itsiopoulos provides 80 delicious recipes, eating plans and nutritional advice, as well as sharing the evidence as to why this diet is the gold standard of healthy eating.

Sustainable, satisfying and suitable for the whole family, this is a diet for life, one that celebrates the pleasures of food as much as it promotes long-term good health and wellbeing.

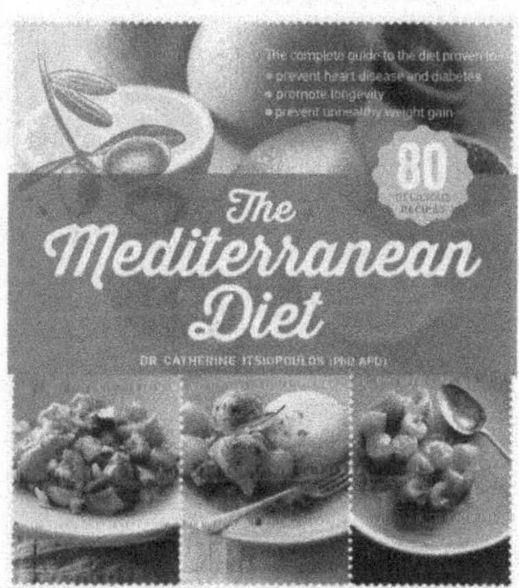

Lola Berry

THE 20/20 DIET COOKBOOK

Leading Australian nutritionist Lola Berry devised the simple yet groundbreaking 20/20 Diet based on her own personal weight journey and many years' experience helping people to shed excess kilos.

In *The 20/20 Diet Cookbook*, Lola shows you how simple it is to eat real foods that are as close to their natural state as possible: unprocessed, nutritious, seasonal and delicious. From breakfasts, smoothies and juices to nourishing snacks, mains and desserts, Lola shares her passion for fresh, healthy food in her own inimitable, charming style. More than a hundred of her favourite recipes are included, such as Roast Chicken with Quinoa, Pistachio and Cranberry Stuffing, Banoffee Pie, moreish Crispy Kale Chips, Strawberry and Almond Pancakes, Mango, Avocado and Macadamia Salad and dreamy Raw Rose and Raspberry Tart.

It's never been so easy to eat and feel well.

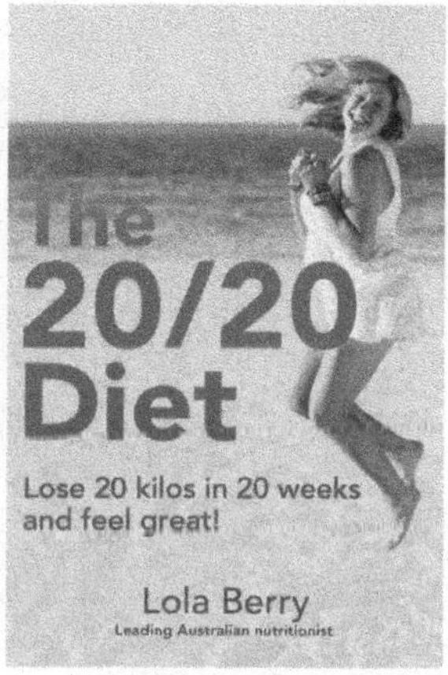